HIV/AIDS - CONTEMPORARY CHALLENGES

Edited by **Nancy Dumais**

HIV/AIDS - Contemporary Challenges
http://dx.doi.org/10.5772/63251
Edited by Nancy Dumais

Contributors

Sphiwe Madiba, Ashraf Alqaqa, Oscar Labra, Daniel Thomas, Pius Tanga, Tomoko Omiya, Yoshihiko Yamazaki, Megumi Shimada, Kazuko Ikeda, Seiko Ishiuchi-Ishitani, Katsumi Ohira, Flavia Kiweewa Matovu, Brian Wigdahl, Michael Nonnemacher, Tiisetso J. Makatjane

Published by InTech
Janeza Trdine 9, 51000 Rijeka, Croatia

Publishing Process Manager Iva Lipovic
Technical Editor SPi Global
Cover InTech Design team

First published February, 2017
Printed in Croatia
Legal deposit, Croatia: National and University Library in Zagreb

Additional hard copies can be obtained from orders@intechopen.com

HIV/AIDS - Contemporary Challenges, Edited by Nancy Dumais
p. cm.
Print ISBN 978-953-51-2961-5
Online ISBN 978-953-51-2962-2

For EU product safety concerns:
IN TECH d.o.o., Prolaz Marije Krucifikse Kozulić 3, 51000 Rijeka, Croatia,
info@intechopen.com or visit our website at intechopen.com.

Meet the editor

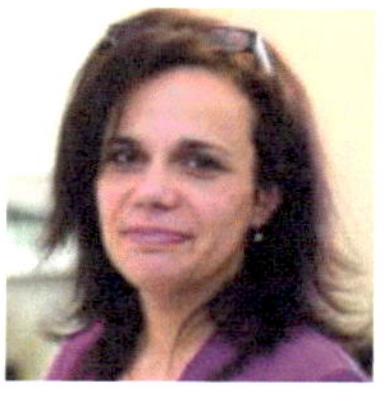

Dr. Nancy Dumais is a Professor of Virology at Université de Sherbrooke, Canada. She received her Diploma (M.Sc.) in Cellular and Molecular Biology and her Doctorate (Ph.D.) in Virology, in 1996 and 2001, respectively, both from Université Laval in Canada. Then, she was a Postdoctoral Researcher at McMaster University where she studied mucosal immunization against HIV. Her research interests include chemokines and chemokines receptors in HIV-1 pathogenesis and cell migration Her laboratory also investigates the roles of prostaglandins in HIV transcription and replication. Also, she is interested in scientific and health education. She gives lectures in molecular biology, microbiology, and virology at different universities.

Contents

Preface IX

Section 1 Medical Aspects 1

Chapter 1 **Human Immunodeficiency Virus (HIV) Infection and Cancer 3**
Lorena Loarca, Joseph A. Fraietta, Vanessa Pirrone, Zsofia Szep and Brian Wigdahl

Chapter 2 **HIV-Associated Vasculopathy 43**
Ashraf Alqaqa

Chapter 3 **Anti-Retroviral–Based HIV Pre-Exposure Prophylaxis for Women: Recent Advances and Next Steps 55**
Flavia Matovu Kiweewa, Kenneth K. Mugwanya and Francis Kiweewa

Section 2 Social and Economic Aspects 65

Chapter 4 **Three Decades of HIV/AIDS Pandemic: Challenges Faced by Orphans in Tembisa, South Africa 67**
Pius Tangwe Tanga, Princess Khumalo and Priscilla Gutura

Chapter 5 **Difficulties and Coping Strategies Experienced by Employed People with HIV in Japan: A Qualitative Study Comparing High and Low Sense of Coherence Groups 83**
Tomoko Omiya, Yoshihiko Yamazaki, Megumi Shimada, Kazuko Ikeda, Seiko Ishiuchi-Ishitani and Katsumi Ohira

Chapter 6 **The Contextual Environmental Factors Shaping Disclosure of HIV Status across Populations Groups in Sub-Saharan Africa 105**
Sphiwe Madiba

Chapter 7 **The Persistence of Stigma Linked with HIV/AIDS in Health-Care Contexts: A Chronic Social Incapacity 125**
Oscar Labra and Daniel Thomas

Chapter 8 **Economic Globalization, HIV and AIDS and Gender Dimensions in the Lesotho Textiles and Garment Industry 141**
Pius Tangwe Tanga, Haruna M. Bello, Tiisetso J. Makatjane and Tumelo Tsikoane

Preface

Over 36.7 million people worldwide are infected with human immunodeficiency virus type 1 (HIV-1). Also, over 2.1 million new cases are diagnosed each year with half of these infections occurring in individuals younger than 25 years (UNAIDS, 2016). Fortunately, with increasing efficacy of antiretroviral therapy, HIV/AIDS has shifted from a disease with high mortality to a chronic illness with substantial longevity. Nevertheless, the continuing pandemic reminds us that despite the unrelenting quest for knowledge since the early 1980s, many challenges remain for the development of efficient treatment and vaccines. Moreover, people living with HIV/AIDS still face many problems, and this book proposes to explore some of them.

The book is divided into two intertwined sections. The first section examines medical aspects of HIV/AIDS and is composed of three chapters. The first chapter is a comprehensive update on HIV-1 infection and cancer. Indeed, HIV-1 infection confers an increased risk for the development of many types of cancer. In this chapter, the authors provide a better understanding of HIV-1–induced oncogenesis. Also, they explore viral mechanisms of immune perturbation, as well as nonimmune microenvironmental abnormalities that lead to oncogenesis. They also discuss how outcomes of therapy will provide the basis for better diagnosis and management of cancer. In addition to cancer, people living with HIV/AIDS have an increased rate of vasculopathy. Thus, Chapter 2 is a comprehensive review of HIV-related vasculopathy and provides basic and clinical knowledge that will be useful to manage the pathology and improve patient care successfully. Chapter 3 is a review of recent advances in the development of new biomedical interventions and findings from pivotal clinical trials. This chapter sheds light on future-generation HIV prevention strategies for women.

The second section of the book is a compendium of chapters dedicated to social and economic aspects of HIV/AIDS. Chapter 4 discusses the challenges faced by orphans of HIV and AIDS regarding health, shelter, education and food. Chapter 5 examines the range of difficulties HIV-positive individuals experience and their coping strategies, especially in the workplace. Disclosure of HIV-positive status is a public health intervention strategy to reduce HIV infections and improve HIV treatment and care. Disclosure has both potential benefits and risks for both the individual and society. However, HIV stigma is still present. Chapter 6 investigates the contextual environmental factors shaping disclosure of HIV status across population groups in sub-Saharan Africa, while Chapter 7 provides an analysis of the stigmatisation of people living with HIV/AIDS within healthcare contexts. Finally, Chapter 8 discusses how the global economic crisis, as well as HIV and AIDS, poses threat to the industry in South Africa.

I am privileged to be the editor of such meaningful book, and I am grateful to all the authors and researchers who contribute to the content of this book. This book describes in detail many challenges that people living with HIV/AIDS face, and I hope that the information provided in this book will be of great interest not only to graduate students but also to active academics and practitioners.

Dr. Nancy Dumais
Université de Sherbrooke,
Canada

Section 1

Medical Aspects

Chapter 1

Human Immunodeficiency Virus (HIV) Infection and Cancer

Lorena Loarca, Joseph A. Fraietta, Vanessa Pirrone,
Zsofia Szep and Brian Wigdahl

Additional information is available at the end of the chapter

http://dx.doi.org/10.5772/67162

Abstract

Human immunodeficiency virus type 1 (HIV-1) infection confers an increased risk for the development of many cancers. Although the incidences of acquired immunodeficiency syndrome (AIDS)-defining malignancies have declined since the advent of antiretroviral therapy (ART), a number of non-AIDS–defining cancers appear more common in HIV-1–infected individuals relative to the general population. ART-treated HIV-1–infected subjects are also aging, leading to an increased cancer burden in these populations. However, longevity alone is not sufficient to explain these epidemiologic trends. A causative link between HIV-1–induced immune suppression and elevated cancer risk is well defined in certain malignancies; however, the direct role of HIV-1 replication products in oncogenesis remains unclear. Nevertheless, it is evident that cooperation between HIV-1 and co-infecting viruses in targeting immune compartments as well as nonimmune microenvironments can regulate both the development and progression of cancer. Treating cancer in HIV-1–infected patients remains challenging due to drug interactions, compounded side effects and intensified immunosuppression from chemotherapy and/or radiation. While survival of HIV-1–infected patients with certain cancers now rivals that of their uninfected counterparts, a better understanding of HIV-1–induced oncogenesis, viral mechanisms of immune perturbation, nonimmune microenvironmental abnormalities and outcomes of therapy will provide the basis for better diagnosis and management of cancer.

Keywords: HIV-1, cancer, non-AIDS–defining cancer, AIDS-defining cancer, coinfection

1. Introduction

The acquired immune deficiency syndrome (AIDS) caused by chronic infection with the human immunodeficiency virus type 1 (HIV-1) leads to severe immunosuppression and death from immunologic and neurologic dysfunction as well as a number of opportunistic infections if left untreated. Prior to the introduction of anti-retroviral therapy (ART), the risk of AIDS patients developing Kaposi's sarcoma (KS), non-Hodgkin's lymphoma (NHL) and cervical cancer was enhanced by several fold. These three cancers have been referred to as AIDS-defining cancers (ADCs). Since 1996, when ART became readily available, the incidence of ADCs dramatically decreased and this was attributed to the partial restoration of immune function [1]. With the HIV-1–infected patient population now living longer, however, these individuals exhibit an increased risk of developing other types of cancers that are referred to as non-AIDS–defining cancers (NADCs) [2]. NADCs can be classified as either virus or nonvirus related. Although many of these cancers are directly linked to HIV-1 infection, many are not. Several factors have been associated with the elevated number of cases of NADCs observed in the last couple of decades, including low $CD4^+$ T-cell counts, chronic inflammation, tobacco usage, alcohol exposure, long-term ART exposure, advanced age and co-infection with oncogenic viruses. Some of the viruses associated with the development of NADCs include human papillomavirus (HPV), Epstein-Barr virus (EBV), human T-cell leukemia virus type 1 (HTLV-1), hepatitis B virus (HBV) and hepatitis C virus (HCV).

Several lines of evidence have established an association between chronic HIV-1 infection and the development of cancer. In this review, we examine the epidemiology, etiology and pathological characteristics of cancer in the setting of chronic HIV-1 infection. We also discuss the direct participation of HIV-1 proteins such as the transactivator of transcription (Tat) protein and the envelope glycoprotein (gp)120 in potentiating tumorigenesis as well as cooperation between HIV-1 and co-infecting viruses in inducing cell transformation. In addition, we discuss the interactions between HIV-1 and immune as well as nonimmune microenvironments and their involvement in driving oncogenesis and cancer progression. Finally, challenges to the management of cancer in HIV-1–infected patients will be investigated, with a focus on the development of evidence-based treatment approaches that combine ART with effective cancer treatment plans.

2. Types of cancers observed in HIV-1–infected patients

The success of ART has extended the life span of many HIV-1–infected patients; however, with an improved life span comes an increased risk of developing a number of chronic conditions and malignancies such as cardiovascular disease, neurologic syndromes and cancer [3]. The latter accounts for approximately 25–35% of HIV-1–associated deaths, with lymphoma being the most common cause of cancer among HIV-1–infected individuals [4]. As previously indicated, the cancers that affect these individuals have been generally divided into two main categories: ADCs and NADCs.

2.1. AIDS-defining cancers (non-Hodgkin's lymphoma, Kaposi's sarcoma and cervical cancer)

2.1.1. Non-Hodgkin's lymphoma (NHL)

The Center for Disease Control and Prevention (CDC) classified non-Hodgkin's lymphoma (NHL), Kaposi's sarcoma (KS) and cervical cancer as ADCs. The occurrence of any of these cancers in HIV-1–infected individuals indicates the progression of HIV-1 infection to AIDS [5]. After the introduction of the ART in 1996, a dramatic improvement in immunologic function in HIV-1–infected subjects was observed as well as a rapid decline in the number of AIDS-related deaths [3].

NHL originates from malignant transformation of the precursor and mature forms of B, T and natural killer (NK) cells that mainly migrate to the lymphoid organs and the hematopoietic tissues but also to other organs [6]. There are 35 types of NHL, which can be differentiated based on histology. The CDC initially classified four of these as ADCs, which include diffuse large B cell lymphoma (DLBCL) with centroblastic characteristics, DLBCL with immunoblastic features, primary nervous system lymphoma (PNSL) and Burkitt's lymphoma [1]. In the setting of HIV-1 infection, EBV has been linked to the etiology of NHL [7]. Even though the number of cases of NHL associated with HIV-1 infection initially declined following the introduction of ART, the incidence of NHL in the HIV-1–infected population remains elevated and is 4–23 times higher than uninfected individuals [8]. A study conducted by Achenbach et al. demonstrated that the incidence of NHL remains high even in HIV-1–infected patients on ART. For instance, the incidence of NHL in HIV-1–infected individuals with HIV-1 viral loads of 51–500 RNA copies/ml and those individuals with $CD4^+$ T-cell counts >200 cells/μl remains elevated. By the year 2000, NHL accounted for 11% of deaths among HIV-1–infected individuals and that number had only decreased by 1% five years later [8].

A study conducted by Gopal et al. established the mortality and predictive indicators of death in a cohort of 23,050 HIV-1–infected patients from 1996 to 2010. Of the total patients enrolled in this study, 476 patients developed lymphoma, of which 79 patients were diagnosed with Hodgkin's lymphoma (HL), 201 patients with DLBCL, 54 patients with PNSL and the remaining 86 patients were diagnosed with other types of NHL. Furthermore, in 223 patients, lymphoma appeared despite ART. The 5-year survival rate was 50% for patients with BL, 44.1% for those with DLBCL, 22.8% for those with primary brain lymphoma and 43.3% of patients with other types of NHL. The overall identification of risk factors for mortality included increased age, lymphoma diagnosis while on ART, a low $CD4^+$ T-cell count and high viral load [4].

Another study in which results from a number of AIDS registries was linked to several cancer registries demonstrated that there were differences in the clinical presentation of NHL pre- and post-ART. In the pre-ART era (1983–1995), 33% and 38% of patients were presented with intermediate- and high-grade systemic NHL, respectively. Following the introduction of ART, the percentage of patients with intermediate-grade NHL increased to 49%, whereas the percentage of patients with high-grade NHL decreased to 19% [9]. Additionally, the survival rate of patients with systemic NHL increased significantly in the post-ART era relative to the pre-ART era, with a rise from 4 months as seen pre-ART to 9 months post-ART. There was also a change in the proportion of patients who had NHL of CNS origin, with a decrease from 28% pre-ART to 17% post-ART. However, this decrease in incidence did not correlate with an increase in survival rate [9].

2.1.2. Kaposi's sarcoma (KS)

KS is a neoplasm that arises from mesenchymal cells at multiple foci and involves the recruitment of inflammatory cells, malignant transformation of endothelial cells and neoangiogenesis

[10]. In the context of HIV-1 infection, KS development is linked to co-infection with human herpes virus 8 (HHV-8). The formation of KS lesions is associated with immunosuppression, reactivation of a latent HHV-8 infection and activation of the immune response [11]. Before the onset of the AIDS pandemic, KS was a very rare cancer. In the United States, the incidence of KS between 1973 and 1978 within the white male population was 0.3 per 100,000 person-years. This trend dramatically increased with the onset of the AIDS epidemic, peaking by 1985–1986. It has been estimated that by 1989–1991, the occurrence of KS was 8.9 per 100,000 person-years [1]. Between 1990 and 1995, KS was the most prevalent AIDS-defining cancer in the United States. During this time, HIV-1–infected individuals were at a 53,000 fold-increased risk of developing KS compared to the general population [1]. Following the introduction of ART, however, the incidence of KS decreased considerably due to three factors: (i) decreased HIV-1 replication; (ii) improvement in the HHV-8-specific immune response; and (iii) the angiogenesis inhibitory effects associated with protease inhibitors used to treat HIV-1 infection [12]. Accordingly, the immune status of patients plays a large role in the development of KS. In fact, patients who developed KS while on ART began with low CD4 counts and usually developed KS within 6 months of beginning therapy [13]. Other studies have also shown that while ART did decrease the risk of KS, those who proceeded to develop KS while on ART exhibited evidence of virologic failure [14]. These collective observations underscore the important link between decreased immune function due to HIV-1 infection and the development of KS.

2.1.3. Cervical cancer

Cervical cancer is a neoplastic condition that originates in the cervix. In 1993, invasive cervical cancer began to be included as an AIDS-defining diagnosis. Epidemiological evidence suggests that the precursor lesions, cervical intraepithelial neoplasia, or squamous intraepithelial lesion occur more frequently in women with HIV-1 [15]. In HIV-1–infected females, co-infection with the HPV is associated with invasive cervical cancer. Notably, it is estimated that HPV accounts for 70% of all cervical cancer cases [16]. However, not all women living with HPV infection develop cervical cancer. Factors that may influence the development of cervical cancer include a high level of HPV DNA, sustained HPV infection and infection with certain "high-risk" subtypes of HPV, including HPV 16 and 18. In the context of co-infection with HIV-1, a reduced $CD4^+$ T-cell count is associated with an elevated risk of developing cervical cancer [17]. Furthermore, cervical cancer presents in a more aggressive form with a lower survival time in HIV-1–infected women compared to women who are not infected with HIV-1. Even though ART leads to partial restoration of immune function in HIV-1–infected patients, it remains uncertain whether the incidence of cervical cancer among HIV-1–infected women has been affected by ART.

Studies of patient cohorts in which individual subject data concerning ART use were examined have generated conflicting results, with reduced risk attributed to this therapy reported in some but not in all cases [18]. In contrast, other groups have documented an increased risk for developing invasive cervical cancer following the introduction of ART (e.g., relative risk: 1.46 with a 95% confidence interval of 1.09–1.94) [19, 20]. These discordant results could have several explanations including the increased life expectancy of HIV-1–infected female patients and/or inadequate screening programs for these women [21]. Nevertheless, it is evident that ART may not prevent the appearance of invasive cervical cancer as it was previously thought. A more recent study which focused on assessing prevalence and identifying associated risk factors for developing precancerous cervical lesions among HIV-1–infected women in Kenya demonstrated that subjects who were not treated with ART were 2.21 times more likely to present with precancerous lesions than ART patients [22]. Although the mechanisms underlying how ART-mediated immune reconstitution affects HPV-induced lesions are unclear, the regular screening of HIV-1–infected women remains critically important. In this regard, the initiation of ART could act as leverage for cancer screening in resource-limited settings [22].

2.2. Non-AIDS-defining cancers: Virus related (EBV, HPV, HBV, HCV, and HTLV-1)

With the improvement in morbidity, mortality and life expectancy linked to the introduction of ART, the incidence of ADCs has declined, whereas the incidence of NADCs has paradoxically increased. Examples of NADCs include lung cancer, hepatocellular carcinoma (HCC), colorectal cancer, anal cancer and Hodgkin's lymphoma (HL) among others [3]. While ADCs have been demonstrated to potentially be associated with viral co-infection (i.e., KS linked to infection with HHV-8), NADCs can also be further categorized as either virus or nonvirus related. Unfortunately, HIV-1–infected patients have an increased risk of exposure and subsequent infection with oncogenic viruses, including hepatitis B and C virus (HBV and HCV), human papillomavirus (HPV), Epstein-Barr virus (EBV) and human T-cell leukemia virus type 1 (HTLV-1). This elevated risk of exposure lies on a continuum with the development of cancer as a direct result of infections with these tumorigenic viruses, even in the post-ART era [23].

2.2.1. Epstein-Barr virus (EBV): Hodgkin's lymphoma (HL)

In individuals not infected with HIV-1, between 20% and 50% of HL cases have been attributed to EBV infection; however, 75–100% of the HL cases observed in HIV-1–infected patients have been etiologically attributed to EBV infection. It has been postulated that aberrant $CD4^+$ T-cell responses specific to EBV in HIV-1–infected patients are risk factors for developing HL [24]. After the introduction of ART, lymphoma became the major cause of cancer-related death in the HIV-1–infected patient population. It was reported in a study of 23,050 HIV-1–infected patients enrolled between 1996 and 2010 that 476 (2.1%) individuals were diagnosed with lymphoma, of which 79 patients (16.6%) developed HL. At the time of diagnosis, the mean age was 42.1 years with a mortality rate for HL reported at 7.9% and a 5-year survival of 61.6% [4].

The incidence of HL may be increasing since the advent of ART [25–32], which is likely due to the improvement in the level of immune function [33]. However, the increased relative risk of HL is lower than that observed for aggressive B-cell lymphoma [33]. Prior to the advent of ART, the prognosis of HIV-1–associated HL was poor, with very few individuals cured of their disease [34]. In accordance with these observations, the importance of ART has been demonstrated in the context of improving responses to chemotherapy and prolonging overall survival [35, 36]. Furthermore, HIV-1–infected patients with HL who do not respond to ART have poor outcomes resembling those of the pre-ART era [36]. Additional retrospective and prospective clinical results strongly imply that HIV-1–infected patients with HL who are treated with full-dose chemotherapy and concurrent cART have a significantly improved and comparable prognosis as the uninfected population [37, 38]; gradual recovery of immune function occurs over the course of 6–9 months from the completion of treatment [37, 39].

2.2.2. *Chronic viral hepatitis (HBV and HCV): Hepatocellular carcinoma (HCC)*

It is estimated that 480–540 million people worldwide are currently affected by chronic viral hepatitis. Of these individuals, 350–370 million are infected with HBV and 130–170 million with HCV [40]. In the United States, approximately 25% and 10% of HIV-1–infected persons are co-infected with HCV and HBV, respectively. HCC, a malignancy that arises from hepatocytes, is the fifth leading cause of cancer-related deaths worldwide. An excess of alcohol consumption and viral hepatitis caused by infection with HBV or HCV are the main etiological factors of HCC [41]. In chronic HIV-1 infection, the development of HCC is mainly associated with co-infection with HBV and HCV [42]. Furthermore, liver diseases account for 50% of the mortality in the HIV-1–infected patient population, representing one of the three major causes of non-AIDS–associated deaths [41, 43], with HCC remaining the second leading cause of death in these people [42].

HIV-1 infection increases the risk of developing HCC by seven fold [44]. Indeed, HIV-1 co-infection with HBV or HCV accelerates the progression of either of these infections to liver cirrhosis and ultimately the induction of HCC [42]. In addition to other complications stemming from co-infection, ART has been linked to hepatotoxicity, the effects of which are exacerbated in patients chronically co-infected with HBV or HCV [42]. Additionally, a recent study demonstrated significant differences in the course of HCC progression between HIV-1–infected individuals co-infected with HBV and/or HCV compared to non-HIV-1 co-infected subjects. For instance, HIV-1–infected individuals were diagnosed with HCC at a younger age relative to HIV-1 seronegative subjects (48.03±7.4 versus 67.54±9.6). Even though the rate of HCC reappearance following treatment was similar in both groups, HIV-1–infected patients were re-treated more times and had shorter overall survival rates than in the absence of HIV-1 infection [45].

2.2.3. *Human papilloma virus (HPV): anal cancer*

Anal cancer rarely occurs in the general population. In contrast, the incidence of anal cancer has been increasing since the introduction of ART in HIV-1–infected patients [3]. The risk of developing anal cancer among HIV-1–infected people is 33- to 222-fold higher compared to their uninfected counterparts [46]. Anal cancer particularly affects men who have sex with men between the ages 45–50 [3]. In addition, there have been reports of HIV-1–infected women with abnormal anal cytology, accompanied by the presence of high-risk HPV types [47, 48]. Squamous cell carcinoma (SCC), which originates from the anal canal, is the most prevalent type of anal cancer and its incidence has increased 96% in men and 39% in women over recent decades [3, 46].

Although not all anal cancers are associated with HPV infection, co-infection with HPV 16 is linked to the pathogenesis of SCC. The prevalence of anal HPV 16 co-infection is three to fivefold higher in HIV-1–infected individuals compared to individuals without HIV-1 infection. Low levels of $CD4^+$ T cells correlate with the persistence of HPV infection and predispose individuals to the formation of premalignant anal lesions. Notably, HIV-1–infected females with a history of cervical disease are at an increased risk for developing high-grade anal intraepithelial neoplasia [48–50]. Progression of these lesions into invasive anal cancer occurs as the life span of HIV-1–infected patient populations has been extended due to ART [3]. Screening and treatment protocols are not yet well established for these types of malignancies, which underscore the need for research on anal HPV-associated disease, particularly in the setting of HIV-1 infection.

2.2.4. Human T-cell leukemia virus (HTLV-1): adult T-cell leukemia/lymphoma (ATL and ATLL)

Leukemia is a hematologic cancer characterized by the expansion of immature or abnormal leukocytes [51]. HTLV-1 infects $CD4^+$ T cells, which leads to a malignancy that affects 20 million people worldwide. In less than 5% of the infected patients, HTLV-1 infection can cause adult T-cell leukemia (ATL) or adult T-cell leukemia/lymphoma (ALL) [52]. In the context of HIV-1 infection, co-infection with HTLV-1 is linked to the etiology of leukemia and lymphoma [51]. HIV-1/HTLV-1 co-infection is frequently encountered in areas where HTLV-1 infection is more prevalent, particularly among high risk groups such as intravenous drug users. In areas where HIV-1 infection is high, 10% of HIV-1–infected patients are also co-infected with HTLV-1 [52]. The worldwide incidence of leukemia/lymphoma in individuals co-infected with HIV-1 and HTLV-1 is currently unclear [52]. In a cohort of 21,000 patients residing in the United States, Poiesz et al. studied the prevalence of HTLV-1–induced T-cell lymphoma and found eight patients with lymphoma who tested positive for HTLV-1. One of these patients was also co-infected with HIV-1, presenting with a stage IV lymphoma [53]. In a case study of a 43-year-old African American male with ATL and HIV-1/HTLV-1 co-infection, it was reported that a period of remission after treatment with chemotherapeutic agents and zidovudine was achieved demonstrating, at least in this patient, that co-infection with HIV-1 may not prevent effective cancer treatment [52].

2.3. Non-AIDS-defining cancers: Nonvirus related (lung cancer, colorectal cancer, and prostate cancer)

2.3.1. Lung cancer

Malignant transformation of lung cells results in the development of lung cancer. Lung cancer is responsible for the majority of cancer-related deaths in men and women in the United States. In 2013, approximately 156,176 people in the United States died from lung cancer [54]. Cigarette smoking or the use of other tobacco products is the main cause of lung cancer development in the general population and also in HIV-1–infected patients. Other risk factors for lung cancer among HIV-1–infected patients include immunosuppression, intravenous drug use, the presence of opportunistic lung infections and aging [2]. HIV-1–infected patients exhibit a twofold increased risk of developing lung cancer relative to the general population [3]. Importantly, it has been reported that HIV-1 infection increases the risk of lung cancer development, even in the absence of smoking [55, 56]. The non-small cell lung cancer types account for 80% of the cases of lung cancer in HIV-1–infected patients. In the United States, squamous cell carcinoma, adenocarcinoma and small cell carcinoma collectively account for the most frequent NADC among HIV-1–infected people, preferentially affecting males over females [3].

The clinical presentations of lung cancer in HIV-1–infected patients pre- and post-ART appear to be the same. Lung cancer appears at a younger age (38–49 years) in HIV-1–infected patients as compared to uninfected individuals (68 years) [57, 58]. There are conflicting reports, however, regarding the clinical outcomes of lung cancer in HIV-1–infected versus uninfected subjects. Some studies have shown that the cancer presents more aggressively, with more severe clinical disease course and a shorter overall survival rate in HIV-1–infected patients relative to uninfected individuals [2].

2.3.2. Colorectal cancer

Colorectal cancer is the third most frequently occurring cancer among men and women and the second leading cause of cancer-associated deaths in the United States [59]. The incidence of colorectal cancer among HIV-1–infected patients has been increasing since the introduction of ART [60]. A study conducted by Patel et al. demonstrated that the incidence rate of colorectal cancer among HIV-1–infected individuals from 1992 to 1995 and from 1996 to 1999 was 39.9 and 39.7 per 100,000 person years, respectively. However, this number increased to 66.2 per 100,000 person years from 2000 to 2003. In contrast, the incidence rate of colorectal cancer among the general population was 20.4, 20.5 and 21.2 per 100,000 person years for the same three time frames [60].

A case controlled study of HIV-1–infected patients with colorectal cancer diagnosed from 1994 to 2003 revealed that this malignancy occurred at a younger age in the HIV-1–infected group compared to the general population in the absence of HIV-1 infection [61]. Furthermore, at the time of diagnosis, 90% of the HIV-1–infected patients presented with advanced stage cancer (stage III/IV) compared to 57% in the uninfected group [61]. These observations were confirmed by Berretta et al. who reported differences in the clinical outcome between 27 HIV-1–infected patients and 54 patients with colorectal cancer in the absence of HIV-1 infection studied from 1985 to 2003. This malignancy presented more aggressively in the HIV-1–infected group, as indicated by more advanced disease staging at the time of diagnosis and a shorter survival time as compared to the uninfected patient cohort [44].

The highest incidence of colorectal cancer in the United States is found in African Americans. Even though African Americans represent only 12% of the total population in the United States, these individuals comprise 50% of HIV-1–infected people in this country. Colorectal cancer develops in HIV-1–infected African American at an earlier age compared to the general population. Kumar et al. studied the clinical presentations of colorectal cancer in a retrospective study of 17 HIV-1–infected African Americans and 42 uninfected matched controls. The mean age of colorectal cancer diagnosis in the HIV-1–infected population was 50.70 versus 59.42 years in the control group [62]. Furthermore, 29.4% of the HIV-1–infected patients in this study were diagnosed with colorectal cancer at a younger age (<45 years) versus 6.35% for the control group. At the time of diagnosis, 52.94% of the HIV-1–infected patients and 43.84% of the uninfected controls had already presented with advanced stage colorectal cancer. Interestingly, the survival time was similar for both groups in this study [62].

2.3.3. *Prostate cancer*

Prostate cancer is the second most frequently occurring cancer in men in the United States [63] and will likely affect 6% of these individuals at an age of 60 within the next decade [64]. There are conflicting data, however, regarding the incidence of prostate cancer in the HIV-1–infected patient population. In a retrospective, multi-institutional study of HIV-1–infected patients conducted in the United States from 1996 to 2006, Pantanowitz et al. showed that the mean age for prostate cancer diagnosis in their cohort was 59 years. Additionally, more than half of the patients already presented stage II–IV prostate cancer, with a mean of $CD4^+$ T-cell count of 336 cells/μl and HIV-1 viral load of 17,319 copies/ml. The majority of these patients became long-term survivors after hormonal treatment, radiation and/or prostatectomy [65]. In terms of risk groups, African American men are particularly susceptible to developing prostate cancer. Furthermore, in the setting of HIV-1 infection, it has been reported that prostate cancer might present more aggressive in African American men [66, 67]. A retrospective study of 54 HIV-1–infected males and 1496 uninfected patients with prostate cancer from 2000 to 2011 was conducted to study the clinical presentation and outcome of the cancer between the two groups. In this study, 92% of the HIV-1–infected patients were African American. At the time of cancer diagnosis, 82% of the HIV-1–infected patients were taking ART and the remaining 14% initiated ART after cancer diagnosis. The median age was 60.7 years for the HIV-1–infected patients and 64 years for the general population. In the HIV-1–infected group, the median $CD4^+$ T-cell levels were 391 cells/μl and the viral titers in 76% of these patients were ≤400 copies/ml. At the time of cancer diagnosis, 73 and 14% of the uninfected group presented with cancer stage I/II and stage III/IV, respectively, whereas 63 and 36% of the HIV-1–infected patient group were categorized as stage I/II and III/IV, respectively. Furthermore, HIV-1 infection was associated with a greater likelihood of presenting with advanced stage cancer at the time of diagnosis as well as greater mortality overall [68].

3. Trends in HIV-1–associated cancers

3.1. Incidence and epidemiology

Prior to the advent of ART, KS and NHL accounted for 99% of all ACDs [69]. Following the introduction of this therapy, however, there was an 84 and 54% decrease in the number of KS and NHL cases, respectively. During this same time period, a 70% reduction in the incidence of all ADCs was observed [25, 69]. Despite this dramatic decline, from 1991–1995 to 2001–2005 when ART was introduced, ADCs continue to be a major problem. For example, more than 2000 cases of ADCs were diagnosed annually in the United States between 2001 and 2005, these cancers were more recently attributed to 15–19% of all deaths in HIV/AIDS patients [70, 71]. As previously stated, one of the most important risk factors for KS and NHL is suppression of the immune system as determined by $CD4^+$ T-cell decline [72–74]. A low $CD4^+$ T-cell count (<50 cells/μl) remains a risk for developing KS, even for HIV-1–infected patients who receive ART [75]. Additional risk factors include advanced age and immune reconstitution inflammatory syndrome resulting from restored immunity to specific infectious or noninfectious antigens following the initiation of ART [76].

In contrast, the frequency of NADCs such as melanoma, HL, anal, prostate and colorectal cancers has been steadily increasing over the past two decades [60]. The overall risk for all NDACs in HIV-1–infected persons is approximately twofold higher than in the general population of the same sex and age [77]. It is estimated that NADCs are currently responsible for 28% of deaths in the HIV-1–infected patient population [12]. Indeed, the frequency of NADCs now exceeds the number of AIDS-defining cancers [78]. Using regression analysis, Coghill et al. established an association between HIV-1 infection and cancer-related mortality of cases reported in six states in the United States from 1996 to 2010. This study included 1,816,461 patients with cancer of whom 6459 were infected with HIV-1 and demonstrated an increased incidence and specific mortality particularly for colorectal, lung and other NDACs [64]. Co-infections with oncogenic viruses account for the largest number of NDACs in HIV-1–infected individuals, but NDACs with a nonviral etiology (e.g., lung cancer) also play an important role. The growing proportion of aged HIV-1–infected individuals, co-infections, immune deficits not controlled by ART and/or risky lifestyle factors place HIV-1–infected subjects at higher risk for developing NDACs compared to the general population [23, 79, 80].

3.2. Risk factors (examples include age, chronic inflammation, immunosuppression, smoking, alcohol use, long-term ART)

HIV-1–infected individuals are exposed to a number of cancer risk factors, including smoking, older age, immunosuppression, viremia and long-term ART (**Figure 1**). It is estimated that in the United States, 50% of HIV-1–infected individuals smoke cigarettes, a 2.5-fold higher prevalence than in the general population [81]. A study conducted by Krishnan et al. identified the risk factors for developing NADCs in a cohort of 3158 treatment-naive HIV-1–infected individuals in the United States who started ART at the initiation of the study. The results indicated that smoking and $CD4^+$ T-cell counts (<350 cells/μl) at study entry were associated with increased risk of developing a NADCs. Anal cancer, basal cell carcinoma, HL and lung cancer were the most common cancers reported in this study [78]. The influence of smoking on cancer development among HIV-1–infected individuals was studied in a Danish cohort of 3503 HIV-1–infected patients and 19,979 matched control subjects. The majority of HIV-1–infeccted patients (77%) had been on ART for a median of 3.3 years at study entry and their median baseline $CD4^+$ T-cell counts were 450 cells/μl. In the HIV-1–infected group, 67% and 76% of patients reported never or actively smoking, respectively, compared to 53% and 39% in the uninfected group. Smoking and virus-associated cancers were most prevalent among HIV-1–infected patients. Indeed, there was a higher risk of developing these types of cancers in the HIV-1–infected group compared to the control population [82]. Furthermore, a recent study showed that HIV-1–infected homosexual male smokers were at higher risk of developing HPV-related anal cancer compared to the nonsmoker control group. Smoking was also associated with higher HPV DNA levels, the development of high-grade anal intraepithelial lesions and anal dysplasia [83].

http://dx.doi.org/10.5772/67162

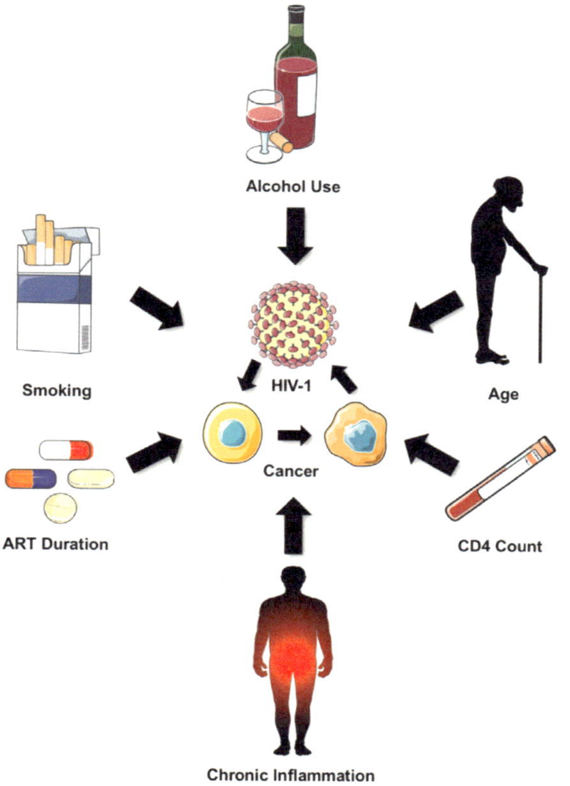

Figure 1. Risk factors for developing cancer in the setting of HIV-1 infection. Factors that may increase the likelihood of developing cancer in HIV-1–infected individuals include alcohol consumption, smoking, the duration of ART, a chronic immunoinflammatory state, CD4 count and/or advanced age. The complex interactions between ART use, HIV-1 replication, aging and other risk factors that are dynamic over time may influence tumor biology in patients with HIV-1 infection.

It has been suggested that the increased number of NADCs in the ART era is due in part to the increased life expectancy following the introduction of this therapy to the HIV-1–infected patient population [12]. A systematic review conducted by Oliveira et al. evaluated the role of ART on the frequency of NADCs among people living with HIV-1. In this study, 21 reports were reviewed, analyzing a total of 2 million person-years and 10,891 new cases of NADCs. The results show that after the introduction of ART, the rate of KS and NHL decreased, whereas the rate of cervical cancer increased. The risk of developing NADCs increased, particularly anal, colorectal, HL, liver, lung and prostate cancers [12].

The role of immunosuppression and viremia in the development of NADCs was evaluated in a cohort of 11,459 HIV-1–infected patients on ART in the Netherlands. Of the total number of patients, 236 patients were diagnosed with NADCs, 102 were infection-related and 134 were not associated with infection. The most common cancer in the infection-related group was anal cancer (37 patients), followed by laryngeal cancer (21) and HCC (16). At the time of cancer diagnosis, the median $CD4^+$ T-cell count was 340 cells/μl (range: 210–540 cells/μl). Furthermore, the longer that a patient spent with a low $CD4^+$ T-cell count (<200 cells/μl), their likelihood of developing an NADC, particularly with infectious etiology increased. Additional risk factors for the development of NADCs in this patient cohort included longevity and developing AIDS before the initiation of ART [84].

A study conducted in Portugal with HIV-1–infected patients showed that the most prevalent NADCs in this group were skin and lung cancers and HCC. KS (32%), NHL (16%) and cervical cancer (4%) accounted for the cases involving ADCs. Importantly, factors such as a longer interval of HIV-1 infection and ART, as well as high $CD4^+$ T-cell counts and HIV type 2 (HIV-2) infection were linked to developing NADCs, whereas impaired immunity, HBV co-infection, cigarette smoking and alcohol consumption were associated with the emergence of ADCs [85].

In a randomized clinical trial of 5472 HIV-1–infected patients, Silverberg et al. studied the effects of discontinuing ART on cancer development. There were two groups of patients studied based on treatment status as continuous ART and discontinuous ART. In the discontinuous ART arm, the treatment was interrupted when the $CD4^+$ T-cell counts were >350 cells/μl and resumed when the counts were <250 cells/μl. Of the total number of patients, 70 developed cancer. There was an increased rate of KS and NHL in the discontinuous ART group, with low $CD4^+$ T-cell counts and the detection of HIV-1 RNA defined as risk factors. According to these variables, the risk of developing NADCs was similar in both groups [86].

The effects of long-term use of ART on cancer development were evaluated in a cohort of 12,872 HIV-1–infected patients who were followed from 1996 to 2008. The incidence of ADC, particularly KS and NHL, decreased as the time on ART increased. This trend was partially attributed to the effects of ART in decreasing HIV-1 RNA levels and restoring $CD4^+$ T cell counts. Interestingly, there was no association between the use of ART and the risk of developing NADCs. However, there was a lower incidence of noninfectious-related NADCs as the ART intervals were increased over time, particularly in the case of prostate cancer [87].

Increased plasma levels of interleukin (IL)-6 and C-reactive protein (CRP), two markers of inflammation, are closely associated with cancer induction. In a prospective study of a cohort of 5023 HIV-1–infected patients, Borges et al. examined the link between the presence of inflammatory factors (IL-6 and CRP) and coagulation markers (e.g., D-dimer) and cancer risk. After a follow up of 24,000 person-years, 172 patients were diagnosed with cancer. The most frequent infection-related malignancies were NHL, HL and anal cancer; the malignancies most often encountered and unrelated to infection were lung, prostate and colorectal cancer. Importantly, there was a significant association between elevated serum levels of IL-6, CR and D-dimer and the risk of cancer development, with high levels of IL-6 exhibiting the strongest correlation [88].

4. Mechanisms of HIV-1–associated cancer

Although an unequivocal link exists between HIV-1 infection and the development of certain cancers, it remains unclear whether HIV-1 acts directly as an oncogenic agent. In the context of

HIV-1 infection, viral-induced tumorigenesis appears to rely on multiple factors, which typically involve cooperation between co-infecting viruses as well as aberrations in immune and nonimmune microenvironments. In this regard, we will describe the mechanisms underlying HIV-1–associated oncogenesis with a focus on both the direct tumor-promoting capacities of viral products on cells and indirect causes of the cooperative induction of cancer that are instead related to the ability of HIV-1 disease to cause profound immune dysregulation. Notably, the importance of viral co-factor cooperation in malignant transformation is underscored in HIV-1–infected individuals due to a high degree of immunodeficiency and/or the chronic immune activation/inflammatory state that increases susceptibility to infection and numerous replicative and oncogenic pathways with multiple tumor viruses [89].

The increased incidence of aggressive B-cell lymphomas in HIV-1–infected subjects compared to individuals with other forms of immune suppression has been documented [90, 91], but remains poorly understood. While this phenomenon may be attributed to the failure of immune surveillance due to direct and bystander T-cell depletion and/or microenvironment changes that define pathogenic HIV-1 infections, it stands to reason that HIV-1 replication products may also contribute to oncogenesis. In further support of this idea, it has been shown that HPV-induced cervical dysplasia and cancer are frequent complications of HIV-1 infection [92–94], with no clear association between occurrence and the degree of host immune suppression [93, 95]. Thus, while this malignancy has been shown to be aggressive, less responsive to treatment and often recurrent in HIV-1–infected women, there appears to be no difference in the severity of neoplasia in asymptomatic patients with HIV-1 infection compared to those who have progressed to AIDS [95]. These collective clinical observations indicate that immunodeficiency may not be the sole mediator of cancer development during the course of HIV-1 disease and implicate a more direct role for HIV-1 with respect to potentiating neoplasia.

The contributions of HIV-1–induced molecular alterations in inducing neoplastic transformation independently of immune system perturbation have been demonstrated, primarily through the use of *in vitro* cell line models. In the context of KS, a direct cooperative role of HIV-1 in mediating tumorigenesis has been observed. In a cell line model derived from a primary effusion lymphoma (PEL), HIV-1 infection triggers reactivation of Kaposi's sarcoma herpesvirus (KSHV) or HHV-8 and this effect was the direct action of the HIV-1 transactivator protein Tat [96]. Tat has been shown to be released from HIV-1–infected cells and may bind to and enter uninfected cells, including endothelial cells through its protein transduction domain [97–99]. Tat-mediated signaling has been shown to promote endothelial cell migration and matrix invasion *in vitro* as well as angiogenesis *in vivo* [100–103]. In addition, human KS cells grow more aggressively in HIV-1 Tat transgenic $CD4^+$ T-cell depleted mice compared to nontransgenic control animals [104], although the direct role of Tat in KS development remains controversial [105]. Furthermore, when HIV-1 and KSHV genomes are present in the same cellular environment, bilateral positive transcription of genes from both viruses has been observed. Notably, HIV-1 Tat and Vpr independently activate KSHV transcription, whereas the KSHV KIE2 protein induces activation of HIV-1 LTR-driven transcription [106]. Finally, it has been suggested that by regulating a number of cellular targets, HIV-1 Tat may be involved in altering DNA repair in host cells, potentially leading to genomic instability which may give rise to mutations and contribute to oncogenesis [107]. In particular, Tat induces expression of the DNA polymerase beta gene, which codes for a central mediator in the DNA base-excision repair pathway [108]; HIV-1 Tat has also been implicated in playing a direct role in double-strand break DNA repair, as cellular extracts containing Tat possess a reduced capacity to re-join linearized DNA [109]. These observations may explain at least in part why HIV-1 and KSHV co-infected individuals possess a higher risk for developing KS.

As mentioned earlier in this review, similar to KS, NHL in AIDS patients is associated with another co-infecting virus, in this case, EBV. While current evidence suggests that the chronic immunoinflammatory state associated with HIV-1 disease contributes to B cell activation and ultimately to lymphomagenesis, HIV-1 replication products may also directly contribute to lymphoma induction. HIV-1 envelope protein gp120 has the ability to directly activate B cells through its interaction with DC-SIGN, leading to immunoglobulin gene class-switch recombination, interleukin secretion and activation-induced cytidine deaminase (AID) expression [110]. Because the HIV-1 envelope interfaces with a number of cellular proteins with diverse functions including adhesion molecules, major histocompatibility complex (MHC) components as well as macrophage, B- and T-cell surface proteins, it would be interesting to determine which of these constituents contribute(s) to B-cell activation and consequential lymphomagenesis [111]. It has also been demonstrated that Tat alters the proliferative capacity and apoptosis sensitivity of EBV-immortalized cell lines, suggesting that cells expressing Tat may have a selective growth advantage, thereby potentially giving rise to clones with enhanced oncogenicity [112]. An interaction between HIV-1 Tat and the pRb2/p130 oncosuppressor protein has also been observed, but the effects of Tat on the cell cycle are conflicting, which may be attributed to its dose- as well as cell type-dependent activities [113–115].

Viral cooperativity in the potentiation of cancer induction may involve more than two agents. In fact, one of the most relevant examples of this type of viral cooperation exists between HIV-1, EBV and KSHV in promoting the development of PEL, a prototypic lymphoma that arises in EBV and KSHV co-infected tumor cells in HIV-1–infected patients [116]. Reciprocal molecular interactions between EBV and KSHV promote each other latency in PEL cells, which may contribute to the establishment and maintenance of tumors [117]. Because HIV-1 can induce KSHV transcription (i.e., through Tat and Vpu) and EBV as well as KSHV replication products (EBNA-2 [118] and ORF45 [119], respectively) activate the HIV-1 LTR, viral cooperation appears to be a potential mechanism underlying lymphomagenesis in this setting.

As previously indicated, the occurrence of HPV-induced cervical cancer is independent of immune suppression, unlike a number of other AIDS-associated neoplasms. However, the molecular underpinnings of a more aggressive malignancy in HIV-1–infected women with cervical cancer are poorly understood. In this regard, HIV-1 Tat has been shown to increase the expression of HPV E6 and E7 oncoproteins [120, 121]; the E6-p53 interaction and E7-Rb complex formation result in functional inactivation and aberrant cell cycle control, which is a critical regulator of HPV-induced cervical carcinogenesis [122]. Rb and its family members such as pRb2/p130 may be affected by HIV-1 expression; HIV-1 Tat may block pRb2/p130 mRNA expression, but it is unclear whether or not Tat changes the architecture of the pRb2/p130-E7 interaction [123]. Furthermore, HIV-1 Tat expression has been shown to decrease the mRNA levels of cyclin-dependent kinase inhibitors p21 and p17 [123] that have been implicated in the control of the G_0/G_1 transition and are inactivated by the HPV E7 protein [124, 125]. However, the end result in cervical carcinogenesis and disease progression of these Tat-induced oncogene and tumor suppressor changes remains unclear.

The tumor microenvironment includes a number of immune cellular components, including activated T cells, B cells and macrophages. Over the past several years, the importance of HIV-1 interactions within the microenvironment has gained increasing recognition. HIV-1 disease results in a profound perturbation of cytokine/chemokine levels, which facilitates the development of antiviral immunity as previously reviewed [126]. However, these mediators can also have a detrimental effect on the host by limiting the development of potent immune responses elicited against infection [127] and directly or indirectly affecting cancer development. In fact, studies of cytokines in HIV-1–infected patients were among the earliest reports of aberrant cytokine levels being associated with lymphoma risk [128, 129]. Elevated levels of IL-6, IL-10, CXCL13 and TNFα are associated with increased risk for the development of NHL in HIV-1–infected individuals [128–131]. The induction of pro-inflammatory mediators by HIV-1 infection likely alters the elaboration of other immunomodulatory factors, thus influencing cellular proliferation, apoptosis sensitivity and other physiologic functions associated with the microenvironment [89].

HIV-1–dependent skewing from T helper (h)1 to Th2 $CD4^+$ T-cell subpopulations has been considered an important step in immune dysregulation as previously reviewed [132]. Increased Th2 differentiation likely precedes the development of AIDS-related NHL and may also play a role in Th17 upregulation [111]. Th17 cells are present in the microenvironment of a number of different murine and human tumors [133]. Furthermore, in the context of AIDS-NHL pathogenesis, Th2 or Th17 cytokines are known to drive AID expression [134].

The dysregulation of cytokine/chemokine pathways in the HIV-1–infected patient may also promote neoangiogenesis. In addition to the aforementioned role of Tat in stimulating capillary formation [135], the HIV-1 matrix protein, p17, has been shown to promote angiogenesis through a different mechanism involving the ligation of chemokine receptors [136]. More specifically, the release of p17 from HIV-1–infected cells binds to CXCR1, which subsequently drives human monocytes into the microenvironment in an IL-8 chemokine-like manner resulting in sustained inflammation [137]. Increased levels of IL-6 and TNFα in the plasma of HIV-1–infected patients can induce COX-2 and PGE_2 synthesis, which have been linked to the development of AIDS-related cervical cancer [138], an effect that could be related to the promotion of angiogenesis [139, 140]. The precise role of HIV-1–driven angiogenic mechanisms in the development and progression of cancer has not been elucidated and warrants further investigation.

Finally, the nonimmune microenvironment may drive the development and/or progression of AIDS-related cancers and this may also involve mechanisms of viral cooperation [89]. In lymphomas, the nonimmune microenvironment is largely composed of endothelia, stromal cells and fibroblasts that contribute to tumorigenicity. In AIDS-associated NHLs, studies on nonimmune microenvironmental components have focused on neoangiogenesis, although it is presently debated whether HIV-1 may influence this process through productive infection of endothelial cells [89]. Interestingly, Liapis et al. recently demonstrated that the amount of neovasculature was consistently increased in AIDS-NHL compared to sporadic NHLs. In these patients, AIDS-NHL microvessel density in virus-infected tissue was directly correlated with EBV expression [135]. While neovascular abnormality may be considered a common process observed in a number of viral diseases, the identification of biomarkers in nonimmune microenvironments and the precise mechanisms of viral oncogenesis in these settings may prove to be important in the diagnosis and management of HIV-1–associated lymphomas.

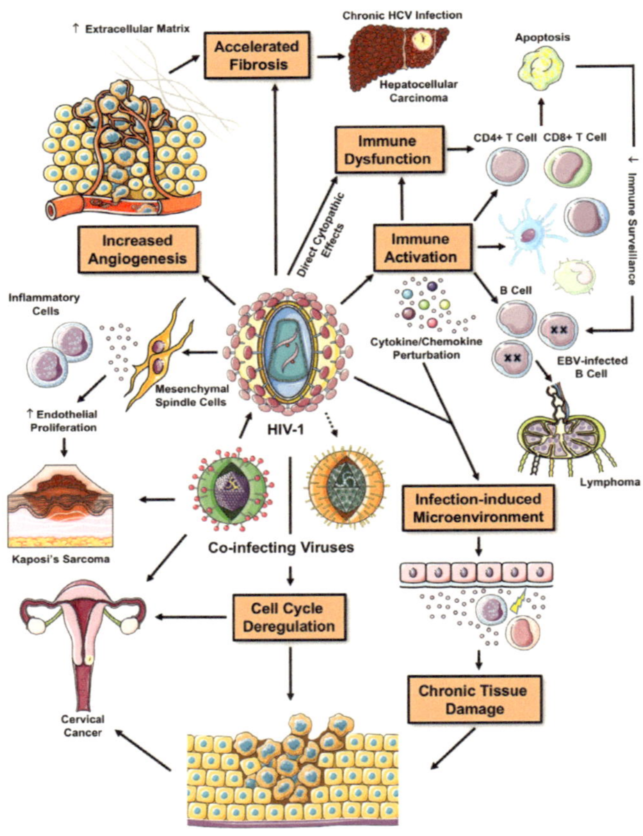

Figure 2. Mechanisms of HIV-1–associated cancer. Increased oncogenesis in the setting of HIV-1 disease usually involves co-infection with other viruses and immune dysfunction, accompanied by decreased immune surveillance. Persistent immune activation as a consequence of HIV-1 infection may lead to chronic tissue damage and the formation of infection-induced microenvironments that potentiate cancer induction. HIV-1 and its products may also influence oncogenesis (usually in the context of viral cooperativity) independently of immune suppression through cell cycle deregulation and/or influencing the nonimmune microenvironment (e.g., increased extracellular matrix, pro-fibrogenic factors and blood vessel formation).

The mechanistic underpinnings of HIV-1 co-infection in accelerating the progression of HCC by HCV may be related to direct effects of HIV-1 on activated hepatic stellate cells (HSCs), the primary fibrogenic cell type in the liver. HSCs are permissive for HIV-1 infection, support viral gene expression and are capable of transmitting infectious virus [141]. Other than induction of pro-inflammatory cytokines, productive infection of HSCs promotes fibrogenic collagen I expression [141]. Similarly, exposing hepatocytes to HIV-1 results in increased production of reactive oxygen species (ROS), collagen and tissue inhibitor of metalloproteinase 1 (TIMP1), an effect that is amplified by concurrent HCV exposure [142]. Another proposed way by which HIV-1 promotes fibrosis is through induction of apoptosis in response to envelope proteins [143, 144] and/or expression of tumor necrosis factor-related apoptosis-inducing ligand (TRAIL) and its cognate death receptors DR4 and DR5 [145, 146]. Taken together, an increase in fibrous tissue with the concomitant destruction of liver cells provides the "soil" for development of cancerous nodules following long periods of chronic liver diseases [147–149]. In addition to highly profibrotic proteins and extracellular matrix constituents, characterization of other nonimmune microenvironment components in the context of HIV-1 infection as well as co-infection conditions is required for the elucidation of well-defined pathophysiological pathways to inform mechanism-based approaches directed against HIV/AIDS-related tumors.

Mechanisms of HIV-1–associated oncogenesis and cancer progression are summarized in **Figure 2**.

5. Management of cancer in HIV-1–infected patients

HIV-1–infected individuals with cancer have lower rates of survival relative to individuals not infected with HIV-1 [150]. While this may be attributed to the aggressive nature of malignancies in the setting of HIV-1–driven immune dysfunction, alternative explanations include the decreased efficacy or increased toxicity of cancer therapy [150–152]. In addition, the disparity between HIV-1–infected and uninfected patients following cancer diagnosis could potentially be a consequence of inadequate cancer treatment due to a survival decrement [153]. Indeed, many HIV-1–infected patients are excluded from clinical trials of cancer therapies and this may contribute to the lack of evidence-based strategies for the management of these patients, especially if treatments are perceived to have diminished effectiveness and/or enhanced toxicity in the background of HIV-1 infection [154].

The absence of cancer treatment for HIV-1–infected participants in a recent study with colon cancer, DLBCL and non-small-cell lung cancer further underscores treatment disparities and raises concern, particularly considering the curative potential of therapy for early-stage cancer [154]. Reduced treatment rates of cancer in the HIV-1–infected population may also be attributed to the limited experience of healthcare providers in managing these cases. Ideal cancer therapy regimens for individuals on ART remain unknown due to a lack of published data to guide clinical decision-making. Furthermore, treatment can be challenging because of drug interactions between antineoplastic agents and antiretrovirals as well as increased immunosuppression from chemotherapy and/or radiation [155, 156]. Notably, some chemotherapeutic agents and ART drugs are metabolized by a similar cytochrome p450 enzyme pathway, which could influence the clearance of these agents and affect toxicity as well as efficacy [157]. Thus, when the concurrent use of ART and radio/chemotherapy is anticipated, overlap in toxicity and drug-drug interactions may influence the optimal choice of cancer treatments [158].

In some cancers, such as DLBCL and anal cancer, results are available to inform the treatment of HIV-1–infected patients [159–163]. Prior to the introduction of ART, low-dose and risk-adapted intensive chemotherapeutic regimens as well as infusional chemotherapy were evaluated for HIV-1–associated NHLs [164, 165]. Outcomes were poor regardless of the type of therapy used and were accompanied by substantial toxicity and the occurrence of opportunistic infections [166–172]. However, since the introduction of ART, a paradigm shift has taken place in the treatment of HIV-1–infected lymphoma patients with survival approaching that of HIV-1–negative subjects [116, 165, 172, 173]. Immunotherapy with anti-CD20 monoclonal antibody (rituximab) and/or standard full-dose chemotherapy can now be safely administered to HIV-1–infected patients in the presence of ART with supportive care including hematopoietic growth factors and prophylaxis for opportunistic infections [173–177]. High-dose chemotherapy and peripheral autologous stem-cell transplantation (ASCT) can be used as salvage therapy in patients with HIV-1 who present with relapsed and refractory lymphoma, including HL [178–183].

Some lymphomas in the setting of HIV-1 infection require special considerations when selecting the most appropriate cancer treatment plan. For example, HIV-1–associated Burkitt lymphoma remains controversial, with the CHOP (cyclophosphamide, doxorubicin, vincristine and prednisone) regimen not currently recommended [175, 184, 185]. The results of small retrospective and phase II clinical trials suggest that intensive chemotherapy for ART-treated Burkitt lymphoma patients with HIV-1 may be acceptable [184, 186, 187].

For other cancers, HIV-1–infected individuals have been largely excluded from clinical trials because they are considered to be vulnerable patients and, therefore, randomized data related to treatment outcomes are unavailable [188]. Nevertheless, case reports and retrospective studies conducted after the introduction of ART have suggested similar treatment toxicity with standard therapy [38, 57, 154, 189–193]. For example, cervical cancer is very common in HIV-1–infected women with an aggressive course and poor treatment outcome [194, 195]. Treatment options for cervical cancer include surgery, radiotherapy and chemotherapy either alone or in combination. In regions with a high prevalence of cervical cancer, the majority of patients receive chemoradiotherapy, which can impair immunity [196]. A number of different therapeutic modalities and modifications have been used to improve outcome of treatment in HIV-1–infected patients with cervical cancer. However, there are no standard guidelines for the management of HIV-1–infected patients diagnosed with cervical cancer and the outcome of standard therapy remains poor. A recent systematic review of cervical cancer management in HIV-1–infected individuals along with their treatment outcomes [197] revealed that patients who started ART early exhibited higher rates of completion of their cancer treatment protocol, suggesting that ART should be commenced early after cervical cancer diagnosis to ensure less toxicity and better compliance with therapy [198–201]. Thus, as it currently stands, HIV-1–infected cervical cancer patients should be managed like their uninfected counterparts [197].

Similarly, recommended treatment options for prostate cancer in HIV-1–infected men are the same as those individuals without HIV-1 infection [191]. Some patients may choose to defer therapy for an extended period of monitoring known as active surveillance. In the ART era, prostate-specific antigen (PSA) kinetics and prostate cancer behavior do not seem to differ between HIV-1–infected and uninfected subjects [191, 202]. Thus, although long-term treatment outcomes in HIV-1–infected patients remain uncertain, these individuals should be offered all screening and treatment options as men in the general population [202].

ART is a main component of treatment for all patients with KS and is an effective anti-KS therapy for approximately 60–70% of patients with limited cutaneous lesions [203–205]. In cases of advanced stage visceral KS or aggressive disease, systemic chemotherapy should be combined with ART. First-line chemotherapy includes combination regimens or pegylated liposomal (L) doxorubicin, which has been shown to be better tolerated [205–207] (with an objective response rate of 59–82%). Second-line chemotherapy consists of low-dose paclitaxel for patients who are resistant to anthracyclines (with an objective response rate of 60–70%) [208]. The emergence of immune reconstitution inflammatory syndrome in ART-treated HIV-1-infected patients, which may lead to the development of KS or accelerate its progression, undoubtedly poses a major challenge to current disease management options [209, 210].

In the era of ART, HIV-1–infected patients with cancer can be treated with more aggressive regimens, including intensive chemotherapy with concomitant stem cell transplants in the case of hematologic malignancies and/or combined chemotherapeutic protocols [116]. Due to the potential risk of adverse drug-drug interactions, the simultaneous use of antineoplastic drugs with antiretroviral agents has been debated [53, 156, 211]. However, contemporary guidelines support the use of ART during chemotherapy [173, 212]. With regard to the management of most HIV-1–associated cancers, treatments that achieve the highest rates of progression-free survival in uninfected individuals are becoming increasingly applicable to HIV-1–infected patients [116]. Nevertheless, additional prospective studies are urgently required to define toxicities associated with the concurrent use of ART and chemotherapy. Such reports should be instrumental in developing evidence-based treatment criteria for these patients [158]. Until this is achieved, healthcare providers should individualize cancer treatment plans (e.g., chemotherapy, surgery, radiation therapy) for HIV-1–infected patients based on laboratory results, the presence of renal or liver dysfunction and the risk of potential drug-related toxicities.

6. Conclusions

Although the management of HIV-1 infection has improved considerably in the last few decades, HIV-1–infected patients are still at high risk compared to the general population, with respect to the development of a spectrum of life-threatening malignancies. There are a number of cancers that present in HIV-1–infected patients at a younger age, more aggressively and with a shorter survival time than a comparable uninfected population. This implies that despite the partial restoration of the immune system in HIV-1–infected patients due to efficacious ART protocols, HIV-1 infection has been identified as a risk factor for the development of cancer, particularly NADCs. Indeed, the oncogenic potential of Tat and gp120 has been examined in various cell lines as well as the cooperation between these proteins with co-infecting viruses to enhance cell transformation. A better understanding of the interactions between HIV-1 and a number of oncogenic viruses in conjunction with immune and nonimmune cells may lead to the development of better therapeutic approaches for the management of cancer in HIV-1–infected patients. Furthermore, there are few randomized studies that have addressed the management of cancer in HIV-1–infected patients. Some of the challenges in the treatment of cancer in HIV-1 infection include increased immunosuppression induced by chemotherapy and/or radiation, as well as the potential for synergistic toxicity caused by antiretrovirals and antioncogenic treatments. Thus, it is imperative that HIV-1–infected patients are included in studies to determine the proper therapeutic approaches that these patients need when diagnosed with cancer.

Author details

Lorena Loarca[1,†], Joseph A. Fraietta[2,3,†], Vanessa Pirrone[4,5,6], Zsofia Szep[5,7] and Brian Wigdahl[4,5,6*]

*Address all correspondence to: bwigdahl@drexelmed.edu

1 Division of Gastroenterology and Hepatology, Mayo Clinic Center for Signaling in Gastroenterology, Mayo Clinic, Rochester, MN, USA

2 Center for Cellular Immunotherapies, University of Pennsylvania, Philadelphia, PA, USA

3 Department of Pathology and Laboratory Medicine, University of Pennsylvania, Philadelphia, PA, USA

4 Department of Microbiology and Immunology, Drexel University College of Medicine, Philadelphia, PA, USA

5 Center for Clinical and Translational Medicine, Institute for Molecular Medicine and Infectious Disease, Drexel University College of Medicine, Philadelphia, PA, USA

6 Sidney Kimmel Cancer Center, Thomas Jefferson University, Philadelphia, PA, USA

7 Division of Infectious Diseases and HIV Medicine, Department of Medicine, Drexel University College of Medicine, Philadelphia, PA, USA

† These authors contributed equally.

References

[1] Blattner WA, Nowak RG. Cancers in People with HIV and AIDS. In: Yarchoan R, editor. Epidemiology of AIDS-Defining Malignancies: Springer: New York; 2014. p. 17–30.

[2] Chiao EY. Epidemiology and Clinical Characteristics of Non-AIDS-Defining Malignancies. In: Dittmer DP, Krown SE, editors. Molecular Basis for Therapy of AIDS-Defining Cancers. Springer: New York; 2010. p. 17–40.

[3] Brugnaro P, Morelli E, Cattelan F, Petrucci A, Panese S, Eseme F, Cavinato F, Barelli A, Raise E. Non-AIDS definings malignancies among human immunodeficiency virus-positive subjects: Epidemiology and outcome after two decades of HAART era. The World Journal of Virology 2015 4:209–218.

[4] Gopal S, Patel MR, Yanik EL, Cole SR, Achenbach CJ, Napravnik S, Burkholder GA, Reid EG, Rodriguez B, Deeks SG, Mayer KH, Moore RD, Kitahata MM, Eron JJ, Richards KL. Temporal trends in presentation and survival for HIV-associated lymphoma in the antiretroviral therapy era. Journal of the National Cancer Institute 2013;105:1221–1229.

[5] Castro KG, Ward JW, Slutsker SL, Buehler JW, Jaffe HW, Berkelman RL. 1993 revised classification system for HIV infection and expanded surveillance case definition for AIDS among adolescents and adults. MMWR Recommendations and Reports 1992;41:1–19.

[6] Krol AD, le Cessie S, Snijder S, Kluin-Nelemans JC, Kluin PM, Noordijk EM. Primary extranodal non-Hodgkin's lymphoma (NHL): the impact of alternative definitions tested in the Comprehensive Cancer Centre West population-based NHL registry. Annals of Oncology. 2003;14(1):131–139.

[7] Ansell SM. Non-Hodgkin lymphoma: Diagnosis and treatment. Mayo Clinic Proceedings 2015;90:1152–1163.

[8] Achenbach CJ, Buchanan AL, Cole SR, Hou L, Mugavero MJ, Crane HM, Moore RD, Haubrich RH, Gopal S, Eron JJ, Hunt PW, Rodriguez B, Mayer K, Saag MS, Kitahata MM; for the Centers for AIDS Research (CFAR) Network of, (CNICS) ICS. HIV viremia and incidence of non-Hodgkin lymphoma in patients successfully treated with antiretroviral therapy. Clinical Infectious Diseases. 2014;58:1599–1606.

[9] Diamond C, Taylor TH, Aboumrad T, Anton-Culver H. Changes in acquired immunodeficiency syndrome-related non-Hodgkin lymphoma in the era of highly active antiretroviral therapy: incidence, presentation, treatment and survival. Cancer. 2006;106(1):128–135. DOI: 10.1002/cncr.21562

[10] Ganem D. KSHV and the pathogenesis of Kaposi sarcoma: listening to human biology and medicine. The Journal of Clinical Investigation. 2010;120(4):939–949. DOI: 10.1172/JCI40567

[11] Robey RC, Bower M. Facing up to the ongoing challenge of Kaposi's sarcoma. Current Opinion in Infectious Diseases 2015;28:31–40.

[12] Cobucci RN, Lima PH, de Souza PC, Costa VV, Cornetta Mda C, Fernandes JV, Goncalves AK. Assessing the impact of HAART on the incidence of defining and non-defining AIDS cancers among patients with HIV/AIDS: A systematic review. Journal of Infection and Public Health. 2015;8:1–10.

[13] Mocroft A, Kirk O, Clumeck N, Gargalianos-Kakolyris P, Trocha H, Chentsova N, Antunes F, Stellbrink HJ, Phillips AN, Lundgren JD. The changing pattern of Kaposi sarcoma in patients with HIV, 1994–2003: the EuroSIDA Study. Cancer. 2004;100(12):2644–2654. DOI: 10.1002/cncr.20309

[14] Portsmouth S, Stebbing J, Gill J, Mandalia S, Bower M, Nelson M, Gazzard B. A comparison of regimens based on non-nucleoside reverse transcriptase inhibitors or protease inhibitors in preventing Kaposi's sarcoma. AIDS. 2003;17(11):F17-F22. DOI: 10.1097/01.aids.0000076309.76477.f1

[15] Ellerbrock TV, Chiasson MA, Bush TJ, Sun XW, Sawo D, Brudney K, Wright TC, Jr. Incidence of cervical squamous intraepithelial lesions in HIV-infected women. JAMA. 2000;283(8):1031–1037.

[16] Frazier EL, Sutton MY, Tie Y, McNaghten AD, Blair JM, Skarbinski J. Screening for Cervical Cancer and Sexually Transmitted Diseases Among HIV-Infected Women. Journal of Women's Health. 2016;25:124–132.

[17] Williamson AL. The interaction between human immunodeficiency virus and human papillomaviruses in heterosexuals in Africa. Journal of Clinical Medicine 2015;4:579–592.

[18] Grulich AE. Cancer: the effects of HIV and antiretroviral therapy and implications for early antiretroviral therapy initiation. Curr Opinion in HIV and AIDS. 2009;4(3):183–187. DOI: 10.1097/COH.0b013e328329c5b2

[19] Gingues S, Gill MJ. The impact of highly active antiretroviral therapy on the incidence and outcomes of AIDS-defining cancers in Southern Alberta. HIV Medication. 2006;7 (6):369–377. DOI: 10.1111/j.1468-1293.2006.00395.x

[20] Cobucci RN, Lima PH, de Souza PC, Costa VV, Cornetta Mda C, Fernandes JV, Goncalves AK. Assessing the impact of HAART on the incidence of defining and non-defining AIDS cancers among patients with HIV/AIDS: a systematic review. Journal of Infection and Public Health. 2015;8(1):1–10. DOI: 10.1016/j.jiph.2014.08.003

[21] Dorrucci M, Suligoi B, Serraino D, Tirelli U, Rezza G. Incidence of invasive cervical cancer in a cohort of HIV-seropositive women before and after the introduction of highly active antiretroviral therapy. Journal of Acquired Immune Deficiency Syndromes. 2001;26(4):377–380.

[22] Memiah P, Mbuthia W, Kiiru G, Agbor S, Odhiambo F, Ojoo S, Biadgilign S. Prevalence and risk factors associated with precancerous cervical cancer lesions among HIV-infected women in resource-limited settings. AIDS Research and Treatment 2012;2012:953743. DOI: 10.1155/2012/953743

[23] Deeken JF, Tjen ALA, Rudek MA, Okuliar C, Young M, Little RF, Dezube BJ. The rising challenge of non-AIDS-defining cancers in HIV-infected patients. Clinical Infectious Diseases. 2012;55(9):1228–1235. DOI: 10.1093/cid/cis613

[24] Deeken JF, Tjen-A-Looi A, Rudek MA, Okuliar C, Young M, Little RF, Dezube BJ. The rising challenge of non–AIDS-defining cancers in HIV-infected patients. Clinical Infectious Diseases 2012;55:1228–1235.

[25] Shiels MS, Pfeiffer RM, Gail MH, Hall HI, Li J, Chaturvedi AK, Bhatia K, Uldrick TS, Yarchoan R, Goedert JJ, Engels EA. Cancer burden in the HIV-infected population in the United States. The Journal of the National Cancer Institute. 2011;103(9):753–762. DOI: 10.1093/jnci/djr076

[26] Powles T, Robinson D, Stebbing J, Shamash J, Nelson M, Gazzard B, Mandelia S, Moller H, Bower M. Highly active antiretroviral therapy and the incidence of non-AIDS-defining cancers in people with HIV infection. Journal of Clinical Oncology. 2009;27(6):884–890. DOI: 10.1200/JCO.2008.19.6626

[27] Bedimo RJ, McGinnis KA, Dunlap M, Rodriguez-Barradas MC, Justice AC. Incidence of non-AIDS-defining malignancies in HIV-infected versus noninfected patients in the HAART era: impact of immunosuppression. Journal of Acquired Immune Deficiency Syndromes. 2009;52(2):203–208. DOI: 10.1097/QAI.0b013e3181b033ab

[28] Marin B, Thiebaut R, Bucher HC, Rondeau V, Costagliola D, Dorrucci M, Hamouda O, Prins M, Walker S, Porter K, Sabin C, Chene G. Non-AIDS-defining deaths and immunodeficiency in the era of combination antiretroviral therapy. AIDS. 2009;23(13):1743–1753. DOI: 10.1097/QAD.0b013e32832e9b78

[29] Franceschi S, Lise M, Clifford GM, Rickenbach M, Levi F, Maspoli M, Bouchardy C, Dehler S, Jundt G, Ess S, Bordoni A, Konzelmann I, Frick H, Dal Maso L, Elzi L, Furrer H, Calmy A, Cavassini M, Ledergerber B, Keiser O. Changing patterns of cancer incidence in the early- and late-HAART periods: the Swiss HIV Cohort Study. British Journal of Cancer. 2010;103(3):416–422. DOI: 10.1038/sj.bjc.6605756

[30] Simard EP, Pfeiffer RM, Engels EA. Spectrum of cancer risk late after AIDS onset in the United States. Archives of Internal Medicine. 2010;170(15):1337–1345. DOI: 10.1001/archinternmed.2010.253

[31] Hessol NA, Katz MH, Liu JY, Buchbinder SP, Rubino CJ, Holmberg SD. Increased incidence of Hodgkin disease in homosexual men with HIV infection. Annals of Internal Medicine. 1992;117(4):309–311.

[32] Serraino D, Carbone A, Franceschi S, Tirelli U. Increased frequency of lymphocyte depletion and mixed cellularity subtypes of Hodgkin's disease in HIV-infected patients. Italian Cooperative Group on AIDS and Tumours. European Journal of Cancer. 1993;29A (14):1948–1950.

[33] Kaplan LD. Management of HIV-associated Hodgkin lymphoma: how far we have come. Journal of Clinical Oncology. 2012;30(33):4056–4058. DOI: 10.1200/JCO.2012.44.8373

[34] Jacobson CA, Abramson JS. HIV-associated Hodgkin's lymphoma: Prognosis and therapy in the era of cART. Advances in Hematology 2012;2012:507257. DOI: 10.1155/2012/507257

[35] Gerard L, Galicier L, Boulanger E, Quint L, Lebrette MG, Mortier E, Meignin V, Oksenhendler E. Improved survival in HIV-related Hodgkin's lymphoma since the introduction of highly active antiretroviral therapy. AIDS. 2003;17(1):81–87. DOI: 10.1097/01.aids.0000042593.93174.23

[36] Hoffmann C, Chow KU, Wolf E, Faetkenheuer G, Stellbrink HJ, van Lunzen J, Jaeger H, Stoehr A, Plettenberg A, Wasmuth JC, Rockstroh J, Mosthaf F, Horst HA, Brodt HR. Strong impact of highly active antiretroviral therapy on survival in patients with human immunodeficiency virus-associated Hodgkin's disease. British Journal of Haematology. 2004;125(4):455–462. DOI: 10.1111/j.1365-2141.2004.04934.x

[37] Hentrich M, Berger M, Wyen C, Siehl J, Rockstroh JK, Muller M, Fatkenheuer G, Seidel E, Nickelsen M, Wolf T, Rieke A, Schurmann D, Schmidmaier R, Planker M, Alt J, Mosthaf F, Engert A, Arasteh K, Hoffmann C. Stage-adapted treatment of HIV-associated Hodgkin lymphoma: results of a prospective multicenter study. Journal of Clinical Oncology. 2012;30(33):4117–4123. DOI: 10.1200/JCO.2012.41.8137

[38] Montoto S, Shaw K, Okosun J, Gandhi S, Fields P, Wilson A, Shanyinde M, Cwynarski K, Marcus R, de Vos J, Young AM, Tenant-Flowers M, Orkin C, Johnson M, Chilton D, Gribben JG, Bower M. HIV status does not influence outcome in patients with classical Hodgkin lymphoma treated with chemotherapy using doxorubicin, bleomycin, vinblastine and dacarbazine in the highly active antiretroviral therapy era. Journal of Clinical Oncology. 2012;30(33):4111–4116. DOI: 10.1200/JCO.2011.41.4193

[39] Bower M, Stebbing J, Tuthill M, Campbell V, Krell J, Holmes P, Ozzard A, Nelson M, Gazzard B, Powles T. Immunologic recovery in survivors following chemotherapy for AIDS-related non-Hodgkin lymphoma. Blood. 2008;111(8):3986–3990. DOI: 10.1182/blood-2007-10-115659

[40] Koh HK. Viral Hepatitis: The Secret Epidemic: http://www.hhs.gov/asl/testify/2010/06/t20100617b.html; 2010.

[41] Di Benedetto F, Tarantino G, Ercolani G, Baccarani U, Montalti R, De Ruvo N, Berretta M, Adani GL, Zanello M, Tavio M, Cautero N, Tirelli U, Pinna AD, Gerunda GE, Guaraldi G. Multicenter italian experience in liver transplantation for hepatocellular carcinoma in HIV-infected patients. Oncologist. 2013;18:592–599.

[42] Nunnari G, Berreta M, Pinzone MR, Di Rosa M, Berreta S, Cunsolo G, Malaguarnera M, Cosentino S, De Paoli P, Schnell JM, Cacopardo B. Hepatocellular carcinoma in HIV positive patients. European Review for Medical and Pharmacological Sciences 2012;16:1257–1270.

[43] Mallet V, Vallet-Pichard A, Pol S. The impact of human immunodeficiency virus on viral hepatitis. Liver Int. 2011;31:135–139.

[44] Berretta M, Cappellani A, Di Benedetto F, Lleshi A, Talamini R, Canzonieri V, Zanet E, Bearz A, Nasti G, Lacchin T, Berretta S, Fisichella R, Balestreri L, Torresin A, Izzi I, Ortolani P, Tirelli U. Clinical presentation and outcome of colorectal cancer in HIV-positive patients: a clinical case–control study. Onkologie. 2009;32:319–324.

[45] Berretta M, Garlassi E, Cacopardo B, Cappellani A, Guaraldi G, Cocchi S, De Paoli P, Lleshi A, Izzi I, Torresin A, Di Gangi P, Pietrangelo A, Ferrari M, Bearz A, Berretta S,

Nasti G, Di Benedetto F, Balestreri L, Tirelli U, Ventura P. Hepatocellular carcinoma in HIV-infected patients: check early, treat hard. Oncologist. 2011;16:1258–1269.

[46] Chiao EY, Giordano TP, Richardson P, El-Serag HB. Human immunodeficiency virus–aassociated squamous cell cancer of the anus: Epidemiology and outcomes in the highly active antiretroviral therapy era. Journal of Clinical Oncology. 2008;26:474–479.

[47] Cambou MC, Luz PM, Lake JE, Levi JE, Coutinho JR, de Andrade A, Heinke T, Derrico M, Veloso VG, Friedman RK, Grinsztejn B. Anal human papillomavirus (HPV) prevalences and factors associated with abnormal anal cytology in HIV-infected women in an urban cohort from Rio de Janeiro, Brazil. AIDS Patient Care STDS. 2015;29(1):4–12. DOI: 10.1089/apc.2014.0166

[48] Heard I, Etienney I, Potard V, Poizot-Martin I, Moore C, Lesage AC, Ressiot E, Crenn-Hebert C, Flejou JF, Cubie H, Costagliola D, Darragh TM. High prevalence of anal human papillomavirus-associated cancer precursors in a contemporary cohort of asymptomatic HIV-infected women. Clinical Infectious Diseases. 2015;60(10):1559–1568. DOI: 10.1093/cid/civ049

[49] Ravenda PS, Magni E, Botteri E, Manzotti M, Barberis M, Vacirca D, Trovato CM, Dell'Acqua V, Leonardi MC, Sideri M, Fazio N, Zampino MG. Prognostic value of human papillomavirus in anal squamous cell carcinoma. Cancer Chemother Pharmacol. 2014;74 (5):1033–1038. DOI: 10.1007/s00280-014-2582-x

[50] Williamson AL. The interaction between human immunodeficiency virus and human papillomaviruses in heterosexuals in Africa. Journal of Clinical Medicine. 2015;4(4):579–582.

[51] Whitman AG, Bryan BA, Dyson OF, Patel DK, Ramasamy D, Anantharaman S, Reber AJ, Akula SM. AIDS related viruses, their association with leukemia and Raf signaling. Current HIV Research 2005;3:319–327.

[52] Loarca, L., Sullivan, N., Pirrone, V., and B. Wigdahl. "Leukemia and retroviral disease" in Leukemia – Various Types." (eds), InTech Open, Rijeka, Croatia, 2015. ISBN 978-953-51-4319-2.

[53] Poiesz BJ, Papsidero LD, Ehrlich G, Sherman M, Dube S, Poiesz M, Dillon K, Ruscetti FW, Slamon D, Fang C, Williams A, Duggan D, Glaser J, Gottlieb A, Goldberg J, Ratner L, Phillips P, Han T, Friedman-Kien A, Siegal F, Rai K, Sawitsky A, Sheremata LW, Dosik H, Cunningham C, Montagna R. Prevalence of HTLV-I-associated T-cell lymphoma. American Journal of Hematology 2001;66:32–38.

[54] Group USCSW. United States Cancer Statistics: 1999–2013 Incidence and Mortality Web-based Report. Department of Health and Human Services, Centers for Disease Control and Prevention and National Cancer Institute: Atlanta, USA. 2016.

[55] Engels EA, Brock MV, Chen J, Hooker CM, Gillison M, Moore RD. Elevated incidence of lung cancer among HIV-infected individuals. Journal of Clinical Oncology. 2006;24:1383–1388.

[56] Patel P, Tong T, et al., editors. Incidence of non-AIDS-defining malignancies in the HIV outpatient study (HOPS). 11th Conference on Retroviruses and Opportunistic Infections.

Proceedings of the 11th Conference on Retroviruses and Opportunistic Infections, San Francisco, CA; 2004.

[57] Tirelli U, Spina M, Sandri S, Serraino D, Gobitti C, Fasan M, Sinicco A, Garavelli P, Ridolfo AL, Vaccher E. Lung carcinoma in 36 patients with human immunodeficiency virus infection. The Italian Cooperative Group on AIDS and Tumors. Cancer. 2000;88 (3):563–569.

[58] Ricaurte JC, Hoerman MF, Nord JA, Tietjen PA. Lung cancer in HIV-infected patients: a one-year experience. International Journal of STD & AIDS. 2001;12(2):100–102.

[59] Division of Cancer Prevention and Control, Centers for Disease Control and Prevention (June 2016). Retrieved from: https://www.cdc.gov/cancer/colorectal/statistics/

[60] Patel P, Hanson DL, Sullivan PS, Novak RM, Moorman AC, Tong TC, Holmberg SD, Brooks JT. Incidence of types of cancer among HIV-infected persons compared with the general population in the United States, 1992–2003. Annals of Internal Medicine 2008;148:728–736.

[61] Wasserberg N, Nunoo-Mensah JW, Gonzalez-Ruiz C, Beart RWJ, Kaiser AM. Colorectal cancer in HIV-infected patients: a case control study. International Journal of Colorectal Disease 2007;22:1217–1221.

[62] Kumar A, Shah N, Modi Y, Shaaban HS, DePasquale J, DeBari VA, Yerrabothala S, Maroules M, Guron GK. Characteristics of colorectal cancer in the human immunodeficiency virus-infected African American population. Medical Oncology 2012;29:1773–1779.

[63] Prostate Cancer Statistics: http://www.cdc.gov/cancer/prostate/statistics/index.htm; 2015.

[64] Coghill AE, Shiels MS, Suneja G, Engels EA. Elevated cancer-specific mortality among HIV-infected patients in the United States. Journal of Clinical Oncology. 2015;33:2376–2383.

[65] Pantanowitz L, Bohac G, Cooley TP, Aboulafia D, Dezube BJ. Human immunodeficiency virus-associated prostate cancer: clinicopathological findings and outcome in a multi-institutional study. BJU International 2008;101:1519–1523.

[66] Jones J. African-Americans and prostate cancer: why the discrepancies? The Journal of the National Cancer Institute. 2001;93(5):342–344.

[67] Hoffman RM, Gilliland FD, Eley JW, Harlan LC, Stephenson RA, Stanford JL, Albertson PC, Hamilton AS, Hunt WC, Potosky AL. Racial and ethnic differences in advanced-stage prostate cancer: The Prostate Cancer Outcomes Study. The Journal of the National Cancer Institute. 2001;93(5):388–395.

[68] Riedel DJ, Cox ER, Stafford KA, Gilliam BL. Clinical presentation and outcomes of prostate cancer in an urban cohort of predominantly African-American, HIV-infected patients. Urology. 2015;85:415–422.

[69] Eltom MA, Jemal A, Mbulaiteye SM, Devesa SS, Biggar RJ. Trends in Kaposi's sarcoma and non-Hodgkin's lymphoma incidence in the United States from 1973 through 1998. The Journal of the National Cancer Institute. 2002;94(16):1204–1210.

[70] Antiretroviral Therapy Cohort Collaboration. Causes of death in HIV-1-infected patients treated with antiretroviral therapy, 1996–2006: collaborative analysis of 13 HIV cohort studies. Clin Infect Dis. 2010;50(10):1387–1396. DOI: 10.1086/652283

[71] Rodger AJ, Lodwick R, Schechter M, Deeks S, Amin J, Gilson R, Paredes R, Bakowska E, Engsig FN, Phillips A. Mortality in well controlled HIV in the continuous antiretroviral therapy arms of the SMART and ESPRIT trials compared with the general population. AIDS. 2013;27(6):973–979. DOI: 10.1097/QAD.0b013e32835cae9c

[72] Clifford GM, Polesel J, Rickenbach M, Dal Maso L, Keiser O, Kofler A, Rapiti E, Levi F, Jundt G, Fisch T, Bordoni A, De Weck D, Franceschi S. Cancer risk in the Swiss HIV Cohort Study: Associations with immunodeficiency, smoking and highly active antiretroviral therapy. The Journal of the National Cancer Institute. 2005;97(6):425–432. DOI: 10.1093/jnci/dji072

[73] International Collaboration on HIV and Cancer. Highly active antiretroviral therapy and incidence of cancer in human immunodeficiency virus-infected adults. The Journal of the National Cancer Institute. 2000;92(22):1823–1830.

[74] Frisch M, Biggar RJ, Engels EA, Goedert JJ. Association of cancer with AIDS-related immunosuppression in adults. JAMA. 2001;285(13):1736–1745.

[75] Franceschi S, Maso LD, Rickenbach M, Polesel J, Hirschel B, Cavassini M, Bordoni A, Elzi L, Ess S, Jundt G, Mueller N, Clifford GM. Kaposi sarcoma incidence in the Swiss HIV Cohort Study before and after highly active antiretroviral therapy. British Journal of Cancer. 2008;99(5):800–804. DOI: 10.1038/sj.bjc.6604520

[76] Blattner WA, Nowak RG. Epidemiology of AIDS-Defining Malignancies. In: Yarchoan R, editor. Cancers in People with HIV and AIDS: Progress and Challenges. Springer Science +Business Media, New York 2014. p. 17–30.

[77] Vaccher E, Serraino D, Carbone A, De Paoli P. The evolving scenario of non-AIDS-defining cancers: challenges and opportunities of care. Oncologist. 2014;19(8):860–867. DOI: 10.1634/theoncologist.2014–0024

[78] Krishnan S, Schouten JT, Jacobson DL, Benson CA, Collier AC, Koletar SL, Santana J, Sattler FR, Mitsuyasu R. Incidence of non-AIDS-defining cancer in antiretroviral treatment-naïve subjects after antiretroviral treatment initiation: An ACTG Longitudinal Linked Randomized Trials Analysis. Oncology. 2011;80:42–49.

[79] Engels EA. Non-AIDS-defining malignancies in HIV-infected persons: etiologic puzzles, epidemiologic perils, prevention opportunities. AIDS. 2009;23(8):875–885. DOI: 10.1097/QAD.0b013e328329216a

[80] Silverberg MJ, Chao C, Leyden WA, Xu L, Tang B, Horberg MA, Klein D, Quesenberry CP, Jr., Towner WJ, Abrams DI. HIV infection and the risk of cancers with and without a known infectious cause. AIDS. 2009;23(17):2337–2345. DOI: 10.1097/QAD.0b013e3283319184

[81] Park LS, Hernández-Ramírez RU, Silverberg MJ, Crothers K, Dubrow R. Prevalence of non-HIV cancer risk factors in persons living with HIV/AIDS: a meta-analysis. AIDS. 2016;30:273–291.

[82] Helleberg M, Gerstoft J, Afzal S, Kronborg G, Larsen CS, Pedersen C, Bojesen SE, Nodedestgaard BG, Obel N. Risk of cancer among HIV-infected individuals compared to the background population: impact of smoking and HIV. AIDS. 2014;28:1499–1508.

[83] Wieland U, Hellmich M, Wetendorf J, Potthoff A, Swoboda J, Fuchs W, Brockmeryer N, Pfister H, Kreuter A. Smoking and anal high-risk human papillomavirus DNA loads in HIV-positive men who have sex with men. Indian Journal of Medical Microbiology 2015;305:689–696.

[84] Kesselring A, Gras L, Smit C, van Twillert G, Verbon A, de Wolf F, Reiss P, Wit F. Immunodeficiency as a risk factor for non–AIDS-defining malignancies in HIV-1–infected patients receiving combination antiretroviral therapy. CID. 2011;52.

[85] Fernandes LS. Human immunodeficiency virus and cancer. A population of HIV-infected patients at Hospital de Santa Maria and predictors of cancer. Germs. 2012;2.

[86] Silverberg MJ, Neuhaus J, Bower M, Gey D, Hatzakis A, Henry K, Hidalgo J, Lourtau L, Neaton JD, Tambusi G, Abrams DI. Risk of cancers during interrupted antiretroviral therapy in the SMART study. AIDS. 2007;21:1957–1963.

[87] Chao C, Leyden WA, Xu L, Horberg MA, Klein D, Towner WJ, Quesenberry CP, Abrams DI, Silverberg MJ. Exposure to Antiretroviral Therapy and Risk of Cancer in HIV-infected Persons. AIDS. 2012;26:2223–2231.

[88] Borges ÁH, Silverberg MJ, Wentworth D, Grulich AE, Fätkenheuer G, Mitsuyasu R, Tambussi G, Sabin CA, Neaton JD, Lundgren JD. Predicting risk of cancer during HIV infection: the role of inflammatory and coagulation biomarkers. AIDS. 2013;27:1433–1441.

[89] De Paoli P, Carbone A. Microenvironmental abnormalities induced by viral cooperation: Impact on lymphomagenesis. Seminars in Cancer Biology. 2015;34:70–80. DOI: 10.1016/j.semcancer.2015.03.009

[90] Gaidano G, Carbone A, Dalla-Favera R. Pathogenesis of AIDS-related lymphomas: molecular and histogenetic heterogeneity. The American Journal of Pathology. 1998;152 (3):623–630.

[91] Knowles DM. Immunodeficiency-associated lymphoproliferative disorders. Modern Pathology: an official journal of the United States and Canadian Academy of Pathology, Inc. 1999;12(2):200–217.

[92] Sitas F, Pacella-Norman R, Carrara H, Patel M, Ruff P, Sur R, Jentsch U, Hale M, Rowji P, Saffer D, Connor M, Bull D, Newton R, Beral V. The spectrum of HIV-1 related cancers in South Africa. International Journal of Cancer; Journal international du cancer. 2000;88 (3):489–492.

[93] Tweddel G, Heller P, Cunnane M, Multhaupt H, Roth K. The correlation between HIV seropositivity, cervical dysplasia and HPV subtypes 6/11, 16/18, 31/33/35. Gynecologic Oncology. 1994;52(2):161–164. DOI: 10.1006/gyno.1994.1024

[94] Cappiello G, Garbuglia AR, Salvi R, Rezza G, Giuliani M, Pezzotti P, Suligoi B, Branca M, Migliore G, Formigoni Pomponi D, D'Ubaldo C, Ippolito G, Giacomini G, Benedetto A. HIV infection increases the risk of squamous intra-epithelial lesions in women with HPV infection: an analysis of HPV genotypes. DIANAIDS Collaborative Study Group. International Journal of Cancer; Journal international du cancer. 1997;72(6):982–986.

[95] Maiman M, Fruchter RG, Serur E, Remy JC, Feuer G, Boyce J. Human immunodeficiency virus infection and cervical neoplasia. Gynecologic Oncology. 1990;38(3):377–382.

[96] Merat R, Amara A, Lebbe C, de The H, Morel P, Saib A. HIV-1 infection of primary effusion lymphoma cell line triggers Kaposi's sarcoma-associated herpesvirus (KSHV) reactivation. International Journal of Cancer; Journal international du cancer. 2002;97(6):791–795.

[97] Ensoli B, Buonaguro L, Barillari G, Fiorelli V, Gendelman R, Morgan RA, Wingfield P, Gallo RC. Release, uptake and effects of extracellular human immunodeficiency virus type 1 Tat protein on cell growth and viral transactivation. Journal of Virology. 1993;67 (1):277–287.

[98] Vendeville A, Rayne F, Bonhoure A, Bettache N, Montcourrier P, Beaumelle B. HIV-1 Tat enters T cells using coated pits before translocating from acidified endosomes and eliciting biological responses. Molecular Biology of the Cell. 2004;15(5):2347–2360. DOI: 10.1091/mbc.E03-12-0921

[99] Wu RF, Gu Y, Xu YC, Mitola S, Bussolino F, Terada LS. Human immunodeficiency virus type 1 Tat regulates endothelial cell actin cytoskeletal dynamics through PAK1 activation and oxidant production. Journal of Virology. 2004;78(2):779–789.

[100] Albini A, Barillari G, Benelli R, Gallo RC, Ensoli B. Angiogenic properties of human immunodeficiency virus type 1 Tat protein. Proceedings of the National Academy of Sciences of the United States of America. 1995;92(11):4838–4842.

[101] Albini A, Soldi R, Giunciuglio D, Giraudo E, Benelli R, Primo L, Noonan D, Salio M, Camussi G, Rockl W, Bussolino F. The angiogenesis induced by HIV-1 tat protein is mediated by the Flk-1/KDR receptor on vascular endothelial cells. Nature Medicine. 1996;2(12):1371–1375.

[102] Mitola S, Soldi R, Zanon I, Barra L, Gutierrez MI, Berkhout B, Giacca M, Bussolino F. Identification of specific molecular structures of human immunodeficiency virus type 1 Tat relevant for its biological effects on vascular endothelial cells. Journal of Virology. 2000;74(1):344–353.

[103] Scheidegger P, Weiglhofer W, Suarez S, Console S, Waltenberger J, Pepper MS, Jaussi R, Ballmer-Hofer K. Signalling properties of an HIV-encoded angiogenic peptide mimicking vascular endothelial growth factor activity. The Biochemical Journal. 2001;353(Pt 3):569–578.

[104] Prakash O, Tang ZY, He YE, Ali MS, Coleman R, Gill J, Farr G, Samaniego F. Human Kaposi's sarcoma cell-mediated tumorigenesis in human immunodeficiency type 1 tat-expressing transgenic mice. The Journal of the National Cancer Institute. 2000;92(9):721–728.

[105] Weiss R, Boshoff C. Addressing controversies over Kaposi's sarcoma. The Journal of the National Cancer Institute. 2000;92(9):677–679.

[106] Huang CC, Liang YC, Hsu KS. Characterization of the mechanism underlying the reversal of long term potentiation by low frequency stimulation at hippocampal CA1 synapses. The Journal of Biological Chemistry. 2001;276(51):48108–48117. DOI: 10.1074/jbc.M106388200

[107] Nunnari G, Smith JA, Daniel R. HIV-1 Tat and AIDS-associated cancer: targeting the cellular anti-cancer barrier? Journal of Experimental & Clinical Cancer Research: CR. 2008;27:3. DOI: 10.1186/1756-9966-27-3

[108] Srivastava DK, Tendler CL, Milani D, English MA, Licht JD, Wilson SH. The HIV-1 transactivator protein Tat is a potent inducer of the human DNA repair enzyme beta-polymerase. AIDS. 2001;15(4):433–440.

[109] Chipitsyna G, Slonina D, Siddiqui K, Peruzzi F, Skorski T, Reiss K, Sawaya BE, Khalili K, Amini S. HIV-1 Tat increases cell survival in response to cisplatin by stimulating Rad51 gene expression. Oncogene. 2004;23(15):2664–2671. DOI: 10.1038/sj.onc.1207417

[110] He B, Qiao X, Klasse PJ, Chiu A, Chadburn A, Knowles DM, Moore JP, Cerutti A. HIV-1 envelope triggers polyclonal Ig class switch recombination through a CD40-independent mechanism involving BAFF and C-type lectin receptors. Journal of Immunology. 2006;176(7):3931–3941.

[111] Epeldegui M, Vendrame E, Martinez-Maza O. HIV-associated immune dysfunction and viral infection: role in the pathogenesis of AIDS-related lymphoma. Immunologic Research. 2010;48(1–3):72–83. 10.1007/s12026-010-8168-8

[112] Colombrino E, Rossi E, Ballon G, Terrin L, Indraccolo S, Chieco-Bianchi L, De Rossi A. Human immunodeficiency virus type 1 Tat protein modulates cell cycle and apoptosis in Epstein-Barr virus-immortalized B cells. Experimental Cell Research. 2004;295(2):539–548. DOI: 10.1016/j.yexcr.2004.01.018

[113] Regulier EG, Reiss K, Khalili K, Amini S, Zagury JF, Katsikis PD, Rappaport J. T-cell and neuronal apoptosis in HIV infection: implications for therapeutic intervention. International Reviews of Immunology. 2004;23(1–2):25–59.

[114] Luker GD, Leib DA. Luciferase real-time bioluminescence imaging for the study of viral pathogenesis. Methods in Molecular Biology. 2005;292:285–296.

[115] Bettaccini AA, Baj A, Accolla RS, Basolo F, Toniolo AQ. Proliferative activity of extracellular HIV-1 Tat protein in human epithelial cells: expression profile of pathogenetically relevant genes. BMC Microbiology. 2005;5:20. DOI: 10.1186/1471-2180-5-20

[116] Carbone A, Vaccher E, Gloghini A, Pantanowitz L, Abayomi A, de Paoli P, Franceschi S. Diagnosis and management of lymphomas and other cancers in HIV-infected patients. Nature Reviews Clinical Oncology. 2014;11(4):223–238. DOI: 10.1038/nrclinonc.2014.31

[117] Xu D, Coleman T, Zhang J, Fagot A, Kotalik C, Zhao L, Trivedi P, Jones C, Zhang L. Epstein-Barr virus inhibits Kaposi's sarcoma-associated herpesvirus lytic replication in

primary effusion lymphomas. Journal of Virology. 2007;81(11):6068–6078. DOI: 10.1128/JVI.02743-06

[118] Scala G, Quinto I, Ruocco MR, Mallardo M, Ambrosino C, Squitieri B, Tassone P, Venuta S. Epstein-Barr virus nuclear antigen 2 transactivates the long terminal repeat of human immunodeficiency virus type 1. Journal of Virology. 1993;67(5):2853–2861.

[119] Karijolich J, Zhao Y, Peterson B, Zhou Q, Glaunsinger B. Kaposi's sarcoma-associated herpesvirus ORF45 mediates transcriptional activation of the HIV-1 long terminal repeat via RSK2. Journal of Virology. 2014;88(12):7024–7035. DOI: 10.1128/JVI.00931-14

[120] Strickler HD, Palefsky JM, Shah KV, Anastos K, Klein RS, Minkoff H, Duerr A, Massad LS, Celentano DD, Hall C, Fazzari M, Cu-Uvin S, Bacon M, Schuman P, Levine AM, Durante AJ, Gange S, Melnick S, Burk RD. Human papillomavirus type 16 and immune status in human immunodeficiency virus-seropositive women. The Journal of the National Cancer Institute. 2003;95(14):1062–1071.

[121] La Ruche G, You B, Mensah-Ado I, Bergeron C, Montcho C, Ramon R, Toure-Coulibaly K, Welffens-Ekra C, Dabis F, Orth G. Human papillomavirus and human immunodeficiency virus infections: relation with cervical dysplasia-neoplasia in African women. International Journal of Cancer; Journal international du cancer. 1998;76(4):480–486.

[122] Wang HL, Lu DW. Detection of human papillomavirus DNA and expression of p16, Rb and p53 proteins in small cell carcinomas of the uterine cervix. The American Journal of Surgical Pathology. 2004;28(7):901–908.

[123] Nyagol J, Leucci E, Onnis A, De Falco G, Tigli C, Sanseverino F, Torriccelli M, Palummo N, Pacenti L, Santopietro R, Spina D, Gichangi P, Muchiri L, Lazzi S, Petraglia F, Leoncini L, Giordano A. The effects of HIV-1 Tat protein on cell cycle during cervical carcinogenesis. Cancer Biology & Therapy. 2006;5(6):684–690.

[124] Polyak K, Kato JY, Solomon MJ, Sherr CJ, Massague J, Roberts JM, Koff A. p27Kip1, a cyclin-Cdk inhibitor, links transforming growth factor-beta and contact inhibition to cell cycle arrest. Genes & Development. 1994;8(1):9–22.

[125] Snyder EL, Meade BR, Dowdy SF. Anti-cancer protein transduction strategies: reconstitution of p27 tumor suppressor function. Journal of Controlled Release : official journal of the Controlled Release Society. 2003;91(1–2):45–51.

[126] Reuter MA, Pombo C, Betts MR. Cytokine production and dysregulation in HIV pathogenesis: lessons for development of therapeutics and vaccines. Cytokine & Growth Factor Reviews. 2012;23(4–5):181–191. DOI: 10.1016/j.cytogfr.2012.05.005

[127] Katsikis PD, Mueller YM, Villinger F. The cytokine network of acute HIV infection: a promising target for vaccines and therapy to reduce viral set-point? PLoS Pathogens. 2011;7(8):e1002055. DOI: 10.1371/journal.ppat.1002055

[128] Breen EC, Boscardin WJ, Detels R, Jacobson LP, Smith MW, O'Brien SJ, Chmiel JS, Rinaldo CR, Lai S, Martinez-Maza O. Non-Hodgkin's B cell lymphoma in persons with acquired immunodeficiency syndrome is associated with increased serum levels

of IL10, or the IL10 promoter −592 C/C genotype. Clinical Immunology. 2003;109 (2):119–129.

[129] Schroeder JR, Saah AJ, Hoover DR, Margolick JB, Ambinder RF, Martinez-Maza O, Breen EC, Jacobson LP, Variakojis D, Rowe DT, Armenian HK. Serum soluble CD23 level correlates with subsequent development of AIDS-related non-Hodgkin's lymphoma. Cancer Epidemiology, Biomarkers & Prevention: a publication of the American Association for Cancer Research, cosponsored by the American Society of Preventive Oncology. 1999;8(11):979–984.

[130] Hussain SK, Zhu W, Chang SC, Breen EC, Vendrame E, Magpantay L, Widney D, Conn D, Sehl M, Jacobson LP, Bream JH, Wolinsky S, Rinaldo CR, Ambinder RF, Detels R, Zhang ZF, Martinez-Maza O. Serum levels of the chemokine CXCL13, genetic variation in CXCL13 and its receptor CXCR5 and HIV-associated non-hodgkin B-cell lymphoma risk. Cancer Epidemiology, Biomarkers & Prevention : a publication of the American Association for Cancer Research, cosponsored by the American Society of Preventive Oncology. 2013;22(2):295–307. DOI: 10.1158/1055-9965.EPI-12-1122

[131] Breen EC, Hussain SK, Magpantay L, Jacobson LP, Detels R, Rabkin CS, Kaslow RA, Variakojis D, Bream JH, Rinaldo CR, Ambinder RF, Martinez-Maza O. B-cell stimulatory cytokines and markers of immune activation are elevated several years prior to the diagnosis of systemic AIDS-associated non-Hodgkin B-cell lymphoma. Cancer Epidemiology, Biomarkers & Prevention: a publication of the American Association for Cancer Research, cosponsored by the American Society of Preventive Oncology. 2011;20(7):1303–1314. DOI: 10.1158/1055-9965.EPI-11-0037

[132] Romagnani S, Maggi E. Th1 versus Th2 responses in AIDS. Current Opinion in Immunology. 1994;6(4):616–622.

[133] Kryczek I, Wei S, Zou L, Altuwaijri S, Szeliga W, Kolls J, Chang A, Zou W. Cutting edge: Th17 and regulatory T cell dynamics and the regulation by IL-2 in the tumor microenvironment. Journal of Immunology. 2007;178(11):6730–6733.

[134] Fiorentino DF, Bond MW, Mosmann TR. Two types of mouse T helper cell. IV. Th2 clones secrete a factor that inhibits cytokine production by Th1 clones. The Journal of Experimental Medicine. 1989;170(6):2081–2095.

[135] Liapis K, Clear A, Owen A, Coutinho R, Greaves P, Lee AM, Montoto S, Calaminici M, Gribben JG. The microenvironment of AIDS-related diffuse large B-cell lymphoma provides insight into the pathophysiology and indicates possible therapeutic strategies. Blood. 2013;122(3):424–433. DOI: 10.1182/blood-2013-03-488171

[136] Caccuri F, Giagulli C, Bugatti A, Benetti A, Alessandri G, Ribatti D, Marsico S, Apostoli P, Slevin MA, Rusnati M, Guzman CA, Fiorentini S, Caruso A. HIV-1 matrix protein p17 promotes angiogenesis via chemokine receptors CXCR1 and CXCR2. Proceedings of the National Academy of Sciences of the United States of America. 2012;109(36):14580–14585. DOI: 10.1073/pnas.1206605109

[137] Giagulli C, Caccuri F, Cignarella F, Lougaris V, Martorelli D, Bugatti A, Rusnati M, Dolcetti R, Vitali M, Plebani A, Fiorentini S, Caruso A. A CXCR1 haplotype hampers HIV-1 matrix protein p17 biological activity. AIDS. 2014;28(16):2355–2364. DOI: 10.1097/QAD.0000000000000423

[138] Fitzgerald DW, Bezak K, Ocheretina O, Riviere C, Wright TC, Milne GL, Zhou XK, Du B, Subbaramaiah K, Byrt E, Goodwin ML, Rafii A, Dannenberg AJ. The effect of HIV and HPV coinfection on cervical COX-2 expression and systemic prostaglandin E2 levels. Cancer Prevention Research. 2012;5(1):34–40. DOI: 10.1158/1940-6207.CAPR-11-0496

[139] Tsujii M, Kawano S, Tsuji S, Sawaoka H, Hori M, DuBois RN. Cyclooxygenase regulates angiogenesis induced by colon cancer cells. Cell. 1998;93(5):705–716.

[140] Ben-Av P, Crofford LJ, Wilder RL, Hla T. Induction of vascular endothelial growth factor expression in synovial fibroblasts by prostaglandin E and interleukin-1: a potential mechanism for inflammatory angiogenesis. FEBS Letters. 1995;372(1):83–87.

[141] Tuyama AC, Hong F, Saiman Y, Wang C, Ozkok D, Mosoian A, Chen P, Chen BK, Klotman ME, Bansal MB. Human immunodeficiency virus (HIV)-1 infects human hepatic stellate cells and promotes collagen I and monocyte chemoattractant protein-1 expression: implications for the pathogenesis of HIV/hepatitis C virus-induced liver fibrosis. Hepatology. 2010;52(2):612–622. DOI: 10.1002/hep.23679

[142] Lin W, Wu G, Li S, Weinberg EM, Kumthip K, Peng LF, Mendez-Navarro J, Chen WC, Jilg N, Zhao H, Goto K, Zhang L, Brockman MA, Schuppan D, Chung RT. HIV and HCV cooperatively promote hepatic fibrogenesis via induction of reactive oxygen species and NFkappaB. The Journal of Biological Chemistry. 2011;286(4):2665–2674. DOI: 10.1074/jbc.M110.168286

[143] Munshi N, Balasubramanian A, Koziel M, Ganju RK, Groopman JE. Hepatitis C and human immunodeficiency virus envelope proteins cooperatively induce hepatocytic apoptosis via an innocent bystander mechanism. The Journal of Infectious Diseases. 2003;188(8):1192–1204. DOI: 10.1086/378643

[144] Vlahakis SR, Villasis-Keever A, Gomez TS, Bren GD, Paya CV. Human immunodeficiency virus-induced apoptosis of human hepatocytes via CXCR4. The Journal of Infectious Diseases. 2003;188(10):1455–1460. DOI: 10.1086/379738

[145] Jang JY, Shao RX, Lin W, Weinberg E, Chung WJ, Tsai WL, Zhao H, Goto K, Zhang L, Mendez-Navarro J, Jilg N, Peng LF, Brockman MA, Chung RT. HIV infection increases HCV-induced hepatocyte apoptosis. Journal of Hepatology. 2011;54(4):612–620. DOI: 10.1016/j.jhep.2010.07.042

[146] Zheng SJ, Wang P, Tsabary G, Chen YH. Critical roles of TRAIL in hepatic cell death and hepatic inflammation. The Journal of Clinical Investigation. 2004;113(1):58–64. DOI: 10.1172/JCI19255

[147] Delhaye M, Louis H, Degraef C, Le Moine O, Deviere J, Gulbis B, Jacobovitz D, Adler M, Galand P. Relationship between hepatocyte proliferative activity and liver functional

reserve in human cirrhosis. Hepatology. 1996;23(5):1003–1011. DOI: 10.1053/jhep.1996.v23.pm0008621125

[148] Caillot F, Derambure C, Bioulac-Sage P, Francois A, Scotte M, Goria O, Hiron M, Daveau M, Salier JP. Transient and etiology-related transcription regulation in cirrhosis prior to hepatocellular carcinoma occurrence. World Journal of Gastroenterology. 2009;15(3):300–309.

[149] Sanyal AJ, Yoon SK, Lencioni R. The etiology of hepatocellular carcinoma and consequences for treatment. Oncologist. 2010;15 Suppl 4:14–22. DOI: 10.1634/theoncologist.2010-S4-14

[150] Biggar RJ, Engels EA, Ly S, Kahn A, Schymura MJ, Sackoff J, Virgo P, Pfeiffer RM. Survival after cancer diagnosis in persons with AIDS. Journal of Acquired Immune Deficiency Syndromes. 2005;39(3):293–299.

[151] Brock MV, Hooker CM, Engels EA, Moore RD, Gillison ML, Alberg AJ, Keruly JC, Yang SC, Heitmiller RF, Baylin SB, Herman JG, Brahmer JR. Delayed diagnosis and elevated mortality in an urban population with HIV and lung cancer: implications for patient care. Journal of Acquired Immune Deficiency Syndromes. 2006;43(1):47–55. DOI: 10.1097/01.qai.0000232260.95288.93

[152] Spano JP, Atlan D, Breau JL, Farge D. AIDS and non-AIDS-related malignancies: a new vexing challenge in HIV-positive patients. Part II. Cervical and anal squamous epithelial lesions, lung cancer, testicular germ cell cancers and skin cancers. European Journal of Internal Medicine. 2002;13(4):227–232.

[153] Suneja G, Shiels MS, Melville SK, Williams MA, Rengan R, Engels EA. Disparities in the treatment and outcomes of lung cancer among HIV-infected individuals. AIDS. 2013;27(3):459–468. DOI: 10.1097/QAD.0b013e32835ad56e

[154] Suneja G, Shiels MS, Angulo R, Copeland GE, Gonsalves L, Hakenewerth AM, Macomber KE, Melville SK, Engels EA. Cancer treatment disparities in HIV-infected individuals in the United States. Journal of Clinical Oncology. 2014;32(22):2344–2350. DOI: 10.1200/JCO.2013.54.8644

[155] Antoniou T, Tseng AL. Interactions between antiretrovirals and antineoplastic drug therapy. Clinical Pharmacokinetics. 2005;44(2):111–145. DOI: 10.2165/00003088-200544020-00001

[156] Rudek MA, Flexner C, Ambinder RF. Use of antineoplastic agents in patients with cancer who have HIV/AIDS. The Lancet Oncology. 2011;12(9):905–912. DOI: 10.1016/S1470-2045(11)70056-0

[157] Rubinstein PG, Aboulafia DM, Zloza A. Malignancies in HIV/AIDS: from epidemiology to therapeutic challenges. AIDS. 2014;28(4):453–465. DOI: 10.1097/QAD.0000000000000071

[158] Torres HA, Mulanovich V. Management of HIV infection in patients with cancer receiving chemotherapy. Clinical Infectious Diseases. 2014;59(1):106–114. DOI: 10.1093/cid/ciu174

[159] Kaplan LD, Lee JY, Ambinder RF, Sparano JA, Cesarman E, Chadburn A, Levine AM, Scadden DT. Rituximab does not improve clinical outcome in a randomized phase 3 trial

of CHOP with or without rituximab in patients with HIV-associated non-Hodgkin lymphoma: AIDS-Malignancies Consortium Trial 010. Blood. 2005;106(5):1538–1543. DOI: 10.1182/blood-2005-04-1437

[160] Hocht S, Wiegel T, Kroesen AJ, Berdel WE, Runkel N, Hinkelbein W. Low acute toxicity of radiotherapy and radiochemotherapy in patients with cancer of the anal canal and HIV-infection. Acta Oncologica. 1997;36(8):799–802.

[161] Edelman S, Johnstone PA. Combined modality therapy for HIV-infected patients with squamous cell carcinoma of the anus: outcomes and toxicities. International Journal of Radiation Oncology, Biology, Physics. 2006;66(1):206–211. DOI: 10.1016/j.ijrobp.2006.03.049

[162] Cleator S, Fife K, Nelson M, Gazzard B, Phillips R, Bower M. Treatment of HIV-associated invasive anal cancer with combined chemoradiation. European Journal of Cancer. 2000;36(6):754–758.

[163] Wexler A, Berson AM, Goldstone SE, Waltzman R, Penzer J, Maisonet OG, McDermott B, Rescigno J. Invasive anal squamous-cell carcinoma in the HIV-positive patient: outcome in the era of highly active antiretroviral therapy. Diseases of the Colon and Rectum. 2008;51(1):73–81. DOI: 10.1007/s10350-007-9154-7

[164] Tirelli U, Spina M, Gaidano G, Vaccher E, Franceschi S, Carbone A. Epidemiological, biological and clinical features of HIV-related lymphomas in the era of highly active antiretroviral therapy. AIDS. 2000;14(12):1675–1688.

[165] Mounier N, Spina M, Gisselbrecht C. Modern management of non-Hodgkin lymphoma in HIV-infected patients. British Journal of Haematology. 2007;136(5):685–698. DOI: 10.1111/j.1365-2141.2006.06464.x

[166] Errante D, Tirelli U, Gastaldi R, Milo D, Nosari AM, Rossi G, Fiorentini G, Carbone A, Vaccher E, Monfardini S. Combined antineoplastic and antiretroviral therapy for patients with Hodgkin's disease and human immunodeficiency virus infection. A prospective study of 17 patients. The Italian Cooperative Group on AIDS and Tumors (GICAT). Cancer. 1994;73(2):437–444.

[167] Levine AM, Li P, Cheung T, Tulpule A, Von Roenn J, Nathwani BN, Ratner L. Chemotherapy consisting of doxorubicin, bleomycin, vinblastine and dacarbazine with granulocyte-colony-stimulating factor in HIV-infected patients with newly diagnosed Hodgkin's disease: a prospective, multi-institutional AIDS clinical trials group study (ACTG 149). Journal of Acquired Immune Deficiency Syndromes. 2000;24(5):444–450.

[168] Kaplan LD, Straus DJ, Testa MA, Von Roenn J, Dezube BJ, Cooley TP, Herndier B, Northfelt DW, Huang J, Tulpule A, Levine AM. Low-dose compared with standard-dose m-BACOD chemotherapy for non-Hodgkin's lymphoma associated with human immunodeficiency virus infection. National Institute of Allergy and Infectious Diseases AIDS Clinical Trials Group. The New England Journal of Medicine. 1997;336(23):1641–1648. DOI: 10.1056/NEJM199706053362304

[169] Ratner L, Lee J, Tang S, Redden D, Hamzeh F, Herndier B, Scadden D, Kaplan L, Ambinder R, Levine A, Harrington W, Grochow L, Flexner C, Tan B, Straus D, Consortium AM. Chemotherapy for human immunodeficiency virus-associated non-Hodgkin's lymphoma in combination with highly active antiretroviral therapy. Journal of Clinical Oncology. 2001;19(8):2171–2178.

[170] Mounier N, Spina M, Gabarre J, Raphael M, Rizzardini G, Golfier JB, Vaccher E, Carbone A, Coiffier B, Chichino G, Bosly A, Tirelli U, Gisselbrecht C. AIDS-related non-Hodgkin lymphoma: final analysis of 485 patients treated with risk-adapted intensive chemotherapy. Blood. 2006;107(10):3832–3840. DOI: 10.1182/blood-2005-09-3600

[171] Sparano JA, Lee S, Chen MG, Nazeer T, Einzig A, Ambinder RF, Henry DH, Manalo J, Li T, Von Roenn JH. Phase II trial of infusional cyclophosphamide, doxorubicin and etoposide in patients with HIV-associated non-Hodgkin's lymphoma: an Eastern Cooperative Oncology Group Trial (E1494). Journal of Clinical Oncology. 2004;22(8):1491–1500. DOI: 10.1200/JCO.2004.08.195

[172] Little RF, Pittaluga S, Grant N, Steinberg SM, Kavlick MF, Mitsuya H, Franchini G, Gutierrez M, Raffeld M, Jaffe ES, Shearer G, Yarchoan R, Wilson WH. Highly effective treatment of acquired immunodeficiency syndrome-related lymphoma with dose-adjusted EPOCH: impact of antiretroviral therapy suspension and tumor biology. Blood. 2003;101(12):4653–4659. DOI: 10.1182/blood-2002-11-3589

[173] Barta SK, Xue X, Wang D, Tamari R, Lee JY, Mounier N, Kaplan LD, Ribera JM, Spina M, Tirelli U, Weiss R, Galicier L, Boue F, Wilson WH, Wyen C, Oriol A, Navarro JT, Dunleavy K, Little RF, Ratner L, Garcia O, Morgades M, Remick SC, Noy A, Sparano JA. Treatment factors affecting outcomes in HIV-associated non-Hodgkin lymphomas: a pooled analysis of 1546 patients. Blood. 2013;122(19):3251–3262. DOI: 10.1182/blood-2013-04-498964

[174] Levine AM, Noy A, Lee JY, Tam W, Ramos JC, Henry DH, Parekh S, Reid EG, Mitsuyasu R, Cooley T, Dezube BJ, Ratner L, Cesarman E, Tulpule A. Pegylated liposomal doxorubicin, rituximab, cyclophosphamide, vincristine and prednisone in AIDS-related lymphoma: AIDS Malignancy Consortium Study 047. Journal of Clinical Oncology. 2013;31(1):58–64. DOI: 10.1200/JCO.2012.42.4648

[175] Lim ST, Karim R, Nathwani BN, Tulpule A, Espina B, Levine AM. AIDS-related Burkitt's lymphoma versus diffuse large-cell lymphoma in the pre-highly active antiretroviral therapy (HAART) and HAART eras: significant differences in survival with standard chemotherapy. Journal of Clinical Oncology. 2005;23(19):4430–4438. DOI: 10.1200/JCO.2005.11.973

[176] Lim ST, Karim R, Tulpule A, Nathwani BN, Levine AM. Prognostic factors in HIV-related diffuse large-cell lymphoma: before versus after highly active antiretroviral therapy. Journal of Clinical Oncology. 2005;23(33):8477–8482. DOI: 10.1200/JCO.2005.02.9355

[177] Miralles P, Berenguer J, Ribera JM, Rubio R, Mahillo B, Tellez MJ, Lacruz J, Valencia E, Santos J, Rodriguez-Arrondo F, Pintado V, Grupo de Estudio del SRoSA-RL. Prognosis of AIDS-related systemic non-Hodgkin lymphoma treated with chemotherapy and highly active antiretroviral therapy depends exclusively on tumor-related factors. Journal of Acquired Immune Deficiency Syndromes. 2007;44(2):167–173. DOI: 10.1097/QAI.0b013e31802bb5d0

[178] Re A, Michieli M, Casari S, Allione B, Cattaneo C, Rupolo M, Spina M, Manuele R, Vaccher E, Mazzucato M, Abbruzzese L, Ferremi P, Carosi G, Tirelli U, Rossi G. High-dose therapy and autologous peripheral blood stem cell transplantation as salvage treatment for AIDS-related lymphoma: long-term results of the Italian Cooperative Group on AIDS and Tumors (GICAT) study with analysis of prognostic factors. Blood. 2009;114(7):1306–1313. DOI: 10.1182/blood-2009-02-202762

[179] Diez-Martin JL, Balsalobre P, Re A, Michieli M, Ribera JM, Canals C, Conde E, Rosselet A, Gabriel I, Varela R, Allione B, Cwynarski K, Genet P, Espigado I, Biron P, Schmitz N, Hunter AE, Ferrant A, Guillerm G, Hentrich M, Jurado M, Fernandez P, Serrano D, Rossi G, Sureda A, European Group for Blood and Marrow Transplantation Lymphoma Working Party. Comparable survival between HIV+ and HIV− non-Hodgkin and Hodgkin lymphoma patients undergoing autologous peripheral blood stem cell transplantation. Blood. 2009;113(23):6011–6014. DOI: 10.1182/blood-2008-12-195388

[180] Balsalobre P, Diez-Martin JL, Re A, Michieli M, Ribera JM, Canals C, Rosselet A, Conde E, Varela R, Cwynarski K, Gabriel I, Genet P, Guillerm G, Allione B, Ferrant A, Biron P, Espigado I, Serrano D, Sureda A. Autologous stem-cell transplantation in patients with HIV-related lymphoma. Journal of Clinical Oncology. 2009;27(13):2192–2198. DOI: 10.1200/JCO.2008.18.2683

[181] Krishnan A, Palmer JM, Zaia JA, Tsai NC, Alvarnas J, Forman SJ. HIV status does not affect the outcome of autologous stem cell transplantation (ASCT) for non-Hodgkin lymphoma (NHL). Biology of Blood and Marrow Transplantation: journal of the American Society for Blood and Marrow Transplantation. 2010;16(9):1302–1308. DOI: 10.1016/j.bbmt.2010.03.019

[182] Michieli M, Mazzucato M, Tirelli U, De Paoli P. Stem cell transplantation for lymphoma patients with HIV infection. Cell Transplantation. 2011;20(3):351–370. DOI: 10.3727/096368910X528076

[183] Bayraktar UD, Ramos JC, Petrich A, Gupta N, Lensing S, Moore PC, Reid EG, Aboulafia DM, Ratner L, Mitsuyasu R, Cooley T, Henry DH, Barr P, Noy A. Outcome of patients with relapsed/refractory acquired immune deficiency syndrome-related lymphoma diagnosed 1999–2008 and treated with curative intent in the AIDS Malignancy Consortium. Leukemia & Lymphoma. 2012;53(12):2383–2389. DOI: 10.3109/10428194.2012.697559

[184] Carbone A, Cesarman E, Spina M, Gloghini A, Schulz TF. HIV-associated lymphomas and gamma-herpesviruses. Blood. 2009;113(6):1213–1224. DOI: 10.1182/blood-2008-09-180315

[185] Levine AM. Management of AIDS-related lymphoma. Current Opinion in Oncology. 2008;20(5):522–528. DOI: 10.1097/CCO.0b013e3283094ec7

[186] Galicier L, Fieschi C, Borie R, Meignin V, Daniel MT, Gerard L, Oksenhendler E. Intensive chemotherapy regimen (LMB86) for St Jude stage IV AIDS-related Burkitt lymphoma/leukemia: a prospective study. Blood. 2007;110(8):2846–2854. DOI: 10.1182/blood-2006-10-051771

[187] Wang ES, Straus DJ, Teruya-Feldstein J, Qin J, Portlock C, Moskowitz C, Goy A, Hedrick E, Zelenetz AD, Noy A. Intensive chemotherapy with cyclophosphamide, doxorubicin, high-dose methotrexate/ifosfamide, etoposide and high-dose cytarabine (CODOX-M/IVAC) for human immunodeficiency virus-associated Burkitt lymphoma. Cancer. 2003;98(6):1196–1205. DOI: 10.1002/cncr.11628

[188] Persad GC, Little RF, Grady C. Including persons with HIV infection in cancer clinical trials. Journal of Clinical Oncology. 2008;26(7):1027–1032. DOI: 10.1200/JCO.2007.14.5532

[189] Spano JP, Massiani MA, Bentata M, Rixe O, Friard S, Bossi P, Rouges F, Katlama C, Breau JL, Morere JF, Khayat D, Couderc LJ. Lung cancer in patients with HIV Infection and review of the literature. Medical Oncology. 2004;21(2):109–115. DOI: 10.1385/MO:21:2:109

[190] Vyzula R, Remick SC. Lung cancer in patients with HIV-infection. Lung Cancer. 1996;15(3):325–339.

[191] Wosnitzer MS, Lowe FC. Management of prostate cancer in HIV-positive patients. Nature Reviews Urology. 2010;7(6):348–357. DOI: 10.1038/nrurol.2010.61

[192] Berretta M, Lleshi A, Cappellani A, Bearz A, Spina M, Talamini R, Cacopardo B, Nunnari G, Montesarchio V, Izzi I, Lanzafame M, Nasti G, Basile F, Berretta S, Fisichella R, Schiantarelli CC, Garlassi E, Ridolfo A, Guella L, Tirelli U. Oxaliplatin based chemotherapy and concomitant highly active antiretroviral therapy in the treatment of 24 patients with colorectal cancer and HIV infection. Current HIV Research. 2010;8(3):218–222.

[193] Chapman C, Aboulafia DM, Dezube BJ, Pantanowitz L. Human immunodeficiency virus-associated adenocarcinoma of the colon: clinicopathologic findings and outcome. Clinical Colorectal Cancer. 2009;8(4):215–219. DOI: 10.3816/CCC.2009.n.036

[194] Prabha Devi K, Bindhu Priya N. Conventional Pap Smear Screening in HIV Seropositive Women in South India. Journal of Obstetrics and Gynaecology of India. 2013;63(1):55–58. DOI: 10.1007/s13224-012-0204-2

[195] Massad LS, Seaberg EC, Watts DH, Minkoff H, Levine AM, Henry D, Colie C, Darragh TM, Hessol NA. Long-term incidence of cervical cancer in women with human immunodeficiency virus. Cancer. 2009;115(3):524–530. DOI: 10.1002/cncr.24067

[196] Lissoni P, Meregalli S, Bonetto E, Mancuso M, Brivio F, Colciago M, Gardani G. Radiotherapy-induced lymphocytopenia: changes in total lymphocyte count and in lymphocyte subpopulations under pelvic irradiation in gynecologic neoplasms. Journal of Biological Regulators and Homeostatic Agents. 2005;19(3–4):153–158.

[197] Ntekim A, Campbell O, Rothenbacher D. Optimal management of cervical cancer in HIV-positive patients: a systematic review. Cancer Medicine. 2015;4(9):1381–1393. DOI: 10.1002/cam4.485

[198] Gichangi P, De Vuyst H, Estambale B, Rogo K, Bwayo J, Temmerman M. HIV and cervical cancer in Kenya. International Journal of Gynaecology and Obstetrics: the official organ of the International Federation of Gynaecology and Obstetrics. 2002;76 (1):55–63.

[199] Moodley M, Mould S. Invasive cervical cancer and human immunodeficiency virus (HIV) infection in KwaZulu-Natal, South Africa. Journal of Obstetrics and Gynaecology: the journal of the Institute of Obstetrics and Gynaecology. 2005;25(7):706–710. DOI: 10.1080/01443610500294599

[200] Shrivastava SK, Engineer R, Rajadhyaksha S, Dinshaw KA. HIV infection and invasive cervical cancers, treatment with radiation therapy: toxicity and outcome. Radiotherapy and Oncology: journal of the European Society for Therapeutic Radiology and Oncology. 2005;74(1):31–35. DOI: 10.1016/j.radonc.2004.11.006

[201] Gichangi P, Bwayo J, Estambale B, Rogo K, Njuguna E, Ojwang S, Temmerman M. HIV impact on acute morbidity and pelvic tumor control following radiotherapy for cervical cancer. Gynecologic Oncology. 2006;100(2):405–411. DOI: 10.1016/j.ygyno.2005.10.006

[202] Ong WL, Manohar P, Millar J, Royce P. Clinicopathological characteristics and management of prostate cancer in the human immunodeficiency virus (HIV)-positive population: experience in an Australian major HIV centre. BJU International 2015;116 Suppl 3:5–10. DOI: 10.1111/bju.13097

[203] Bower M, Weir J, Francis N, Newsom-Davis T, Powles S, Crook T, Boffito M, Gazzard B, Nelson M. The effect of HAART in 254 consecutive patients with AIDS-related Kaposi's sarcoma. AIDS. 2009;23(13):1701–1706. DOI: 10.1097/QAD.0b013e32832d080d

[204] Cattelan AM, Calabro ML, Gasperini P, Aversa SM, Zanchetta M, Meneghetti F, De Rossi A, Chieco-Bianchi L. Acquired immunodeficiency syndrome-related Kaposi's sarcoma regression after highly active antiretroviral therapy: biologic correlates of clinical outcome. Journal of the National Cancer Institute Monographs. 2001(28):44–49.

[205] Martin-Carbonero L, Barrios A, Saballs P, Sirera G, Santos J, Palacios R, Valencia ME, Alegre M, Podzamczer D, Gonzalez-Lahoz J, Caelyx KSSG. Pegylated liposomal doxorubicin plus highly active antiretroviral therapy versus highly active antiretroviral therapy alone in HIV patients with Kaposi's sarcoma. AIDS. 2004;18 (12):1737–1740.

[206] Lichterfeld M, Qurishi N, Hoffmann C, Hochdorfer B, Brockmeyer NH, Arasteh K, Mauss S, Rockstroh JK, German Clinical AWG. Treatment of HIV-1-associated Kaposi's sarcoma with pegylated liposomal doxorubicin and HAART simultaneously induces effective tumor remission and CD4+ T cell recovery. Infection. 2005;33(3):140–147. DOI: 10.1007/s15010-005-4099-z

[207] Esdaile B, Davis M, Portsmouth S, Sarker D, Nelson M, Gazzard B, Bower M. The immunological effects of concomitant highly active antiretroviral therapy and liposomal anthracycline treatment of HIV-1-associated Kaposi's sarcoma. AIDS. 2002;16(17):2344–2347.

[208] Tulpule A, Groopman J, Saville MW, Harrington W, Jr., Friedman-Kien A, Espina BM, Garces C, Mantelle L, Mettinger K, Scadden DT, Gill PS. Multicenter trial of low-dose paclitaxel in patients with advanced AIDS-related Kaposi sarcoma. Cancer. 2002;95 (1):147–154. DOI: 10.1002/cncr.10634

[209] Ablanedo-Terrazas Y, Alvarado-De La Barrera C, Reyes-Teran G. Towards a better understanding of Kaposi sarcoma-associated immune reconstitution inflammatory syndrome. AIDS. 2013;27(10):1667–1669. DOI: 10.1097/QAD.0b013e328360106b

[210] French MA. HIV/AIDS: immune reconstitution inflammatory syndrome: a reappraisal. Clinical Infectious Diseases. 2009;48(1):101–107. DOI: 10.1086/595006

[211] Pham PA, Flexner C. Emerging antiretroviral drug interactions. The Journal of Antimicrobial Chemotherapy. 2011;66(2):235–239. DOI: 10.1093/jac/dkq448

[212] Antinori A, Marcotullio S, Ammassari A, Andreoni M, Angarano G, Armignacco O, Carosi G, Cinque P, d'Arminio Monforte A, Di Perri G, Ensoli B, Floridia M, Galli M, Mastroianni C, Matteelli A, Mazzotta F, Moroni M, Pal G, Puoti M, Puro V, Rizzardini G, Sagnelli E, Vella S, Vullo V, Lazzarin A, Italian HIVGWG. Italian guidelines for the use of antiretroviral agents and the diagnostic-clinical management of HIV-1 infected persons. Update 2011. The New Microbiologica. 2012;35(2):113–159.

Chapter 2

HIV-Associated Vasculopathy

Ashraf Alqaqa

Additional information is available at the end of the chapter

http://dx.doi.org/10.5772/66655

Abstract

HIV vasculopathy is a wide range of clinical spectrum related to HIV infection. Increasing longevity of HIV-infected individuals secondary to antiretroviral therapy advancements has resulted in increasing the number of patients with HIV-related vasculopathy. Clinicians need to be aware of the different types of HIV vasculopathy to be able to diagnose and manage the pathology and improve patient care.

Keywords: HIV vasculopathy, vascular disease, carotid disease, aortic aneurysm, peripheral arterial disease, cerebral vasculopathy

1. Introduction

Human immunodeficiency virus (HIV) reduces the immunity of a body, making it vulnerable to opportunistic diseases. HIV was first reported in the USA in 1981, in young homosexual men. The young men were said to have severe opportunistic infections [1]. Two years later the virus was labeled as HIV and acquired immune deficiency syndrome (AIDS), if advanced [2]. A patient is diagnosed with AIDS when their immune system is significantly low, and their CD4 count is <200 cells/μl. The areas most affected with HIV/AIDS-infected persons are the Sub-Saharan regions of Africa. More than 72% of the world's population with HIV live in Africa. According to the 2007 report on HIV/AIDS, the world's total population living with this infection is about 33 million [3]. The burden of the worldwide epidemic of HIV infection continues to increase, especially in the developing world. Third World countries experience a vast financial burden of managing and treating HIV-infected and affected persons with scarce resources. The new advancement of potent antiretroviral therapies has, however, made it possible for more patients to live longer, allowing healthcare providers to witness new clinical manifestations of the chronic HIV infection.

There have been major improvements in novel clinical management in a bid to manage HIV [2]. For instance in 1987, HIV was for the first time linked to vasculopathy, impulsive arteriovenous fistula and arterial occlusive disease or aneurysmal infection [4]. The prevalence of symptomatic vasculitis in HIV patients is about 1% according to recent studies [5]. The chief objective of this review will be to describe the HIV-associated vasculopathies in various parts of the body.

Pathogenecity of HIV, which is associated with vasculopathy, is rather complex and hence not fully comprehended. The complexity is a result of several factors such as inflammatory and immunological response to HIV infections. These factors lead to deleterious and dynamic effects on the endothelial and smooth muscle cells of the blood vessels.

HIV infection results in several interleukins and tumor necrosis factor-α (TNF-α) in response to production of viral proteins by the virus. The HIV-transactivator of transcription protein (*tat*) and viral envelope glycoprotein component (gp120) are believed to induce and mediate the inflammatory responses to vessels. This inflammation consequently results in the production of cytokines and adhesion molecules that interfere with endothelial function. In essence, the viral protein accesses the smooth muscle component of the media layer through CD4 surface receptor. Ultimately, this results into abnormal proliferation of the smooth muscle, and abnormal activation of the coagulation cascade [6–10].

Histological studies show an infiltration of the large vessels surrounded by different inflammatory cells including neutrophils, lymphocytes, monocytes and plasma cells in HIV-infected persons. The infiltration of those cells results in obliterate endarteritis, which is an occlusion of the vessels supplying the vasa vasorum, and leads to ischemia, and necrotic changes of the vessel wall are induced [7–11]. Studies of the biopsy and culture of those aneurysms, however, fail to reveal infectious pathogens.

A murine AIDS model has helped investigate pathogenesis of acquired AIDS. In this model the murine leukemia virus (MuLV) is injected into mice. The mice characteristically develop hypergammaglobulinemia, splenomegaly, lymphadenopathy, T-cell and B-cell functional abnormality. The mice also become highly susceptible to opportunistic infections. The murine AIDS and human AIDS have a lot of similarities regarding immune function alterations. Further clinical progression based on this model and vessel wall animal models has suggested a link between endothelial dysfunction and vasculopathy. It has been found that aortas from infected mice have increased concentrations of ICAM-1 and VCAM-1. Moreover, decrease in their contractile responses and impairment in the endothelium-dependent relaxation are observed.

Pathological findings, conversely, have indicated the thinning of the media layer as a result of the viral infection. In addition, they have indicated a direct viral invasion of the aortic fibroblasts at the level of the adventitia. It has therefore been postulated that an autoimmune destructive process can happen as a result of the similarity in the DNA sequence of the viral glycoprotein and a component of the matrix of the vessel wall. Important to note is that, no strong evidence has been found to support this theory.

It has been postulated that an autoimmune destructive process is possible where there is a DNA sequence of the viral glycoprotein, and a component of the matrix of the vessel wall. This, however, is not fully agreeable as there is lack of strong evidence to support the theory [8–12].

To diagnose HIV-associated vasculopathy, other causes of arterial occlusions and aneurysms have to be eliminated. These are mycotic aneurysms caused by syphilis and tuberculosis. Second, arterial occlusions caused by Takayasu's arteritis, vasculitis, and systemic lupus erythematosus (SLE) and Behcet's disease. Finally, elimination of antiphospholipid antibody syndrome-related aneurysms which make close differentials [13–15].

Recent studies indicate that various symptoms of HIV disease have been affecting almost all body organs. For example, studies in radiological, clinical and postmortem indicated cerebral, cardiac, renal and peripheral vascular pathologies in HIV-infected persons. This chapter will look at different HIV-associated vasculopathies affecting the main organ systems in a body.

2. HIV-associated large vessel aneurysm

The large arteries' condition in HIV-infected persons is not very researched, as it is a rare occurrence. Its pathology is different from atherosclerosis and mycotic aneurysm. It is considered a distinct clinical and pathological entity. It is non-infective vasculopathy, where the microbiological cultures of blood, aneurysm wall and thrombus are negative. Furthermore, the patients with atherosclerotic aneurismal disease are older in comparison to patients with aneurysms related to HIV. HIV-related aneurysm is commonly found in young patients in their 30s [10–14].

While the condition stands to affect any large artery, aneurysms typically affect superficial femoral, carotid and popliteal artery. Aneurysms are not uncommonly found to be multiple and have primarily pseudoaneurysm-like focal saccular transformations. Medical practitioners are therefore advised to screen patients for multiplicity using ultrasound or CT scan with contrast. Leukocytoclastic vasculitis of the vasa vasorum and periadventitial vessels is an important mechanism which weakens the wall of the vessel, and leads to focal disruption of the wall at the position of transmural necrosis. This mainly causes the false impression of aneurysm [9, 10, 13, 14]. The symptoms associated with the aneurysm depend on its location and size. It might be that compressive symptoms in an adjacent organ or structure result in life-threatening hemodynamic instability in case of a rupture. Thromboembolic and venous thrombosis are also likely complications of the aneurysm which have often been reported.

Majority of HIV-infected persons with associated aneurysm have advanced immunosuppressed state. This is usually indicated by abnormally reversed CD4:CD8 ratio. Such patients illustrate an abnormally low CD4 count (a median of about 400 cells/μl only). In addition, if such patients have high globulin level, they exhibit low serum albumin consistently [9–13].

While deciding the management approach of HIV-infected persons with asymptomatic aneurysm, it's important to take into consideration their clinical condition and nutrition status. With this in mind, symptomatic aneurysm lesions should be treated according to the standard guidelines, rules and open surgery standard therapy. The use of endovascular therapy has also gained popularity over the past years. HIV-infected patients should be optimized according to standard practice such as an earlier intervention. Conservative treatment on the other hand would be the best option for patients with advanced HIV/ AIDS. Low albumin (<35 g/l) and CD4 count are both indicators of poor operative outcome. Clinical management should, however, maintain a consistency in administering antiretroviral therapy regardless of CD4 level. This is because such prevalence is indicator of an advanced phase of the condition [8–11, 13, 14].

3. Cerebral vasculopathy

Cerebral vasculopathy in HIV-infected patients is infrequently observed. The disease is believed to be under-diagnosed in most cases according to recent reports. HIV vasculopathy of the central nervous system affects small- to medium-sized blood vessels. The HIV-associated aneurysmal disease is frequently of a fusiform type, and occurs in young adults. This type of aneurysm affects carotids and extracranial vessels mainly. On the other hand, the intracranial aneurysm is a rare discovery and is often observed in children. Some reports have linked the low CD4 counts to increased chances of intracerebral vasculopathy occurrence [11, 12, 15, 16].

The primary pathogenesis of intracerebral vasculopathy is not known. However, various studies have shown that postmortem histological examination indicates damage of the interior elastic lamina and fibrosis. This histological examination has also shown interference of the media along with intimal hyperplasia. The resulting aneurysmal and occlusive patterns of this disease tend to lead to ischemic and/or hemorrhagic complications [10–14].

The pathogenesis of HIV-associated cerebral aneurysms has also been postulated to be a result of immune response to the HIV protein. This occurs, according to various researches, inside the endothelial cell. It has been suggested that the use of antiretroviral therapy may exacerbate the vasculopathy because it can lead to immune reconstitution inflammatory syndrome (IRIS) [15, 16].

A similar theory suggested that an abnormal and significant change in the vascular response to blood flow, which occurs due to changes in circulating cytokines and growth factors, can lead to vascular remodeling. These changes are thought to play a main role in aneurismal dilatation. The production of cytokines and growth factors is believed to be caused by opportunistic infections, which involve the blood vessel endothelial wall, allowing it to abnormally increase. Such repeated infections contribute to an amplified production of elastase, which increases the thickness and fragmentation of the internal elastic lamina. Such changes in the lamina are associated with development of fusiform aneurysms. Because of this suggested association, patients with cerebral aneurysm should be investigated for underlying opportunistic infections [11–13].

4. Carotid disease in HIV patients

Carotid intima-media thickness (IMT) measurement by B-mode high-resolution ultrasound is a noninvasive method of assessing atherosclerosis. It is also a strong predictor of cardiovascular events. IMT is considered in HIV persons to evaluate cardiovascular risk.

The prevalence of carotid atherosclerosis in HIV population varies, and correlates with Framingham risk score (FRS). The higher the FRS, the higher the prevalence. The prevalence is estimated to be 26.6% in the very low-risk group and 76.5% in high-risk group. The carotid IMT of individuals with HIV infection was, on average, 0.04 mm thicker (95% confidence interval; and 0.02–0.06 mm, $p < 0.001$) than that of individuals without HIV infection. Carotid plaque also has been found to be 1.5-fold more frequent in HIV patients in comparison to non-infected persons.

It is believed that the traditional CVD risk factors, in addition to HIV infection factors, play a role in this pathology. However, the role of ART is still not clearly confirmed. There are several studies that have suggested the use of ART as a significant and an independent risk associated with carotid atherosclerosis in HIV-infected patients. Moreover, it has been found that there is a moderate independent association between HIV immunological marker and increased carotid IMT and plaque presence [16, 17].

5. HIV-associated vascular thrombosis

Even though women comprise the highest population of HIV-infected persons in Africa, their male counterparts are said to be more likely to have primary arterial thrombosis. In addition, they are likely to present with late advanced limb ischemia. The pathophysiology of this disease is not well comprehended. Several causes of primary HIV infection-associated thrombosis have been documented. The levels of total proteins and the von Willebrand factor have been found to be increased in such patients. This suggested that endothelial cell dysfunction may play a role, as a predisposing factor for primary thrombosis. Hypercoagulable states associated with the HIV infection, including antiphospholipid antibody syndrome, deficiencies in free protein S, protein C, and antithrombin III, could predispose patients to arterial thrombosis [18, 19].

What is unique about HIV-associated vascular thrombosis is the normality of the arterial tree proximal to the thrombosed arteries by duplex ultrasonography, angiography and macroscopic appearance. Second is the thrombosis of all distal vessels with no demonstrable runoff. Duplex ultrasonography also showed hyperechoic 'spotting' in the arterial wall, the 'string of pearls sign', which has also been observed in patients with HIV-associated arterial aneurysms. Both endothelial dysfunction and coagulation abnormality of the HIV patients were found to correlate with the state of immunosuppression [19, 20].

When managing HIV-associated occlusive vasculopathy, the vascular surgical rules should be followed. Patients having less CD4 count should not be excluded from surgical intervention, since surgical findings show that its success does not depend on CD4 levels. The treatment for primary arterial thrombosis includes surgical thrombectomy with or without thrombolysis. The use of corticosteroid post thrombectomy has been considered previously, although it did not decrease the rethrombosis rate. The treatment modality available unfortunately did not significantly alter the level of amputation. The rate of limb salvage in such cases is about 27%. According to therapy researches, it is clear that therapies do not address the underlying ongoing processes. It's important to note that such studies are only but a few; they are sporadic and reflect individual experiences [19–24].

Venous thrombosis is reported as a complication in HIV-infected patients. It is believed to be a result of disturbance of coagulation process. It is estimated that deep vein thrombosis in HIV-infected patients of up to 5% is attributable to a process of thrombophilia. In addition, protein anticardiolipin antibodies and protein C deficiency have been reported in such patients [25–29].

6. HIV-associated peripheral arterial disease

Peripheral arterial disease is a significant clinical management issue in HIV-infected patients. The disease creates a risk of cardiovascular disease, and is associated with increased morbidity and mortality rate. HIV-infected individuals are believed to have higher prevalence and more severe forms of PAD. Measuring ankle-brachial index (ABI) is the initial noninvasive test to diagnose PAD. It usually correlates to obstructive disease and more than 50% stenosis by angiography in the lower extremity arterial system, if abnormal. Moreover, post-exercise ABI measurement could be used to uncover milder diseases.

Low ABI and high ABI readings have been linked to atherosclerosis and increased cardiovascular events. The exact prevalence of PAD in HIV population is still under-studied and not clearly defined. The studies are not numerous and the existing ones show contradicting results. However, the prevalence is believed to be higher than in normal population and in the range of 9.8–13.9%. High ABI prevalence in HIV patients has risen and is estimated to be in the range of 13.3–19.7%. However, none of the classical vascular risk factors were associated with ABI measurements.

Post-exercise ABI measurement change is suggestive of PAD in HIV-infected patients. It has been reported to range from 10.9% to 26.5%, depending on the criteria used. The exercise test was performed to symptomatic versus asymptomatic HIV-patients. Interestingly, the post-exercise changes in ABI are not associated with traditional atherosclerosis risk factors such as diabetes mellitus, hypertensive disorder and dyslipidemia. Screening for subclinical PAD using post-exercise measurement is encouraged in HIV-infected patients, even when they do not depict symptoms of PAD. PAD has a frequent occurrence in young HIV population and coexists with critical limb ischemia. In HIV-infected patients, there is growing evidence suggesting a high prevalence of PAD and a higher risk of developing severe and accelerated atherosclerosis. PAD in HIV patients is six-fold more than in HIV-negative patients [30–33].

The antiretroviral protease inhibitor induces dyslipidemia, making HIV infection a risk factor for atherosclerosis. HIV causes direct injury to the arterial wall, resulting in the initiation of the inflammatory process. Such inflammations contribute to the development of premature atherosclerosis. Endothelial dysfunction in HIV-infected patients is associated with increasing levels of soluble adhesion molecules, cytokines and procoagulant proteins. The effect of the HIV-associated proteins gp(120)on endothelium have been suggested to cause endothelial dysfunction [25–28, 32, 33]. In addition, PAD in HIV-infected patients can occur even in undetectable viral levels or in absence of severely suppressed immune system. This can be explained by the chronic inflammatory state in HIV patients. PAD, in addition, does not correlate to Framingham risk score in the HIV-infected population [34].

http://dx.doi.org/10.5772/66655

7. HIV and atherosclerotic coronary artery disease

HIV-infected patients live longer since the introduction of ART. It is believed that the risk of atherosclerosis in HIV patients is increased because of associated metabolic disturbances. The coronary disease in such infected individuals is considered distinctive. It is usually more diffuse and is associated with circumferential-intimal thickening, atherosclerotic plaques and abnormal proliferation of the smooth muscle. The muscles with luminal protrusions share several similarities with cardiac transplant vasculopathy [34–38]. Reports have suggested that the most common initial presentation of the HIV patient with CAD is acute myocardial infarction and its mortality can go as high as 24%. In addition, more than 40% test positive to triple vessel disease [39–41].

Coronary artery disease (CAD) is commonly observed in patients who are on ART. During a study conducted on this, HIV-infected patients who were not using ART showed a slight risk of ischemic heart disease. The risk was slightly higher in HIV-infected persons who were on ART. However, during the post-ART period there was a significant increase in the risk of ischemic cardiac disease in the HIV-infected population. The 3-year risk for myocardial infarction was 3.6-fold higher in patients on ART in comparison to those who were not [34, 38–43].

There are numerous metabolic changes that are associated with ART (protease inhibitor in particular). They include impaired glucose metabolism and lipodystrophy as a result of increased insulin insensitivity, and they tend to accelerate the atherosclerosis process. The data regarding nucleoside reverse transcriptase inhibitors, as a risk for CAD, are not very clear. In a D.A.D study, abacavir and didanosine were found to be associated with increased risk of myocardial infarction. Consequently, abacavir has been linked to higher cardiovascular events in first 6 months of the infection. Conversely, other studies could not establish a similar relationship, especially after controlling the traditional cardiovascular risk factors. Furthermore, no link was established in non-nucleoside reverse transcriptase inhibitors and integrase inhibitors as an association with cardiovascular events [20, 44–47].

On one hand, HIV infection has been postulated to independently increase the risk of premature CAD. The mechanism by which the virus can accelerate atherosclerosis is multifactorial and complex. This mechanism involves the activation of inflammatory cells, which changes the immune response in HIV patients. This leads to exposure to a variety of xenoantigens from HIV infection and other viral and bacterial infections. These infections result in the ignition of a continuous inflammatory condition that speeds up atherosclerosis [21, 30, 34].

Endothelial dysfunction is an early marker of atherosclerosis. Endothelial dysfunction has been found in young HIV-infected individuals and has been attributed to increased viral load. HIV affects directly the endothelium function and results in increased levels of prothrombotic plasma markers such as von Willebrand factor, b2 microglobulin and thrombomodulin. In addition, it leads to increased levels of the circulating inflammatory molecules, interleukin 6 and D-dimer.

Prevention of CAD is a cornerstone in clinically managing HIV-infected patients. Careful cardiac screening of individuals who are receiving ART is important. Patients with a history in cardiovascular risk factors stand to benefit from such screening as they are at a higher risk.

Identification of asymptomatic atherosclerotic diseases of the coronaries would help to maximize patients' therapy. By the use of risk stratification tests such as coronary artery calcium score, high sensitivity C-reactive protein and carotid intima-medial thickness, HIV patients with higher risk of cardiovascular events can be identified. This will protect such patients from aggressive risk factors through modification and preventive measures.

Interruption of chronic ART therapy is highly discouraged as it could lead to increase in cardiovascular-associated morbidity and mortality. The SMART study has shown that the risk of cardiovascular morbidity and mortality has increased significantly. This is in patients who were assigned to a CD4 cell count guided therapy arm, as compared to their counter parts with continuous therapy arm. However, no studies or theories support an association of CD4 count and CAD [34, 43].

The conventional cardiovascular risk factors are found to be higher in HIV patients. Patients with smoking habits particularly, experience increased risk of atherosclerosis and increase the prothrombotic state [38, 39]. Controlling and modifying the risk factors and comorbidities is important in managing atherosclerosis. The fasting lipids should be checked before starting ART, and followed up to adjust therapy according to the lipids' value changes. If statin therapy is needed to treat high low-density lipoprotein (LDL) levels, the dose to be used should be identified carefully. This is because the risk of statin drug interaction and possible rhabdomyolysis is higher in HIV patients. PI, ritonavir and some antimicrobial agents inhibit specific cytochrome P450 enzymes, which are important in metabolizing several statins. This is because such agents could increase the toxicity of those drugs. Pravastatin (20–40 mg), low-dose atorvastatin (10 mg) and rosuvastatin (5–10 mg) have been suggested as safe if used with protease inhibitors. Ezetimibe can also be added to statin therapy to achieve target levels of LDL. Fibrates are used to control hypertriglyceridemia, if the concentration is above 500 mg/dL.

8. Pulmonary arterial hypertension

HIV-related pulmonary arterial hypertension (PHT) is estimated to occur in 0.5% of the HIV population. It is usually present with nonspecific symptoms such as dyspnea on exertion, lower extremity edema and fatigue. PHT is considered a poor prognostic finding and it is said to lead to right ventricular dysfunction, therefore significantly increasing the mortality rate.

The pathogenesis of HIV-related PHT is complex and still not very well understood. Factors that are believed to participate in the pathogenesis are related to the viral infection in patients. It is believed that the HIV virus stimulates an immune response, which leads to the release of different cytokines and growth factors. This may include the potent vasoconstrictors, endothelin-1, interleukin 6, tumor necrosis factor and platelet-derived growth factor. These immunological responses result in endothelial damage, intimal fibrosis, and stimulate the proliferation of the smooth muscle and fibroblast of the arterioles. Eventually, the pathological structural changes lead to the formation of plexiform lesion. The lesion is quite similar to those found in PaHTN caused by other factors. More recent evidence suggests that the patient's immunologic response, virus HIV-negative factor (Nef), HIV-transactivator of transcription (Tat) accessory proteins and human herpes virus-8 coinfection, may play an important role to cascade events.

Its prognosis is poor and the reported mortality rate is said to be high. PaHTN in HIV population is an independent predictor of mortality with 1-year survival rate reported to range from 51% to 88%. The severity of HIV infection and CD4 cell count has no apparent correlation with this complication. The effect of highly active antiretroviral therapy regimens on the clinical course is still not well defined and is presently being investigated. However, it has been suggested that long-duration treatment with HAART might reduce mortality rate. Currently the treatment of HIV-PaHTN is similar to that of idiopathic pulmonary arterial hypertension patients. There have been reports of the use of diuretics, anticoagulation, phosphodiesterase V inhibitors and calcium channel blockers to treat HIV-PaHTN. HAART prostacyclin analogs (e.g.epoprostenol and endothelin) and receptor inhibitors (such as bosentan) were found to be effective in reducing the pulmonary arterial pressure in HIV patients. Heart-lung transplantation is the last treatment option in this subgroup of patients [21, 22, 34].

9. Conclusion

HIV-associated vascular diseases is not a common occurrence, even though it is considered to be of significant clinical importance. A comprehensive screening for possible etiology such as co-infections, lymphoproliferative disease, and autoimmune disorders, before other pathological attributions to HIV infection is important for appropriate patients' management. HIV-associated vascular disease can be manifested either as aneurysms or occlusive forms. The two forms of diseases can lead to hemorrhagic or ischemic life-threatening complications, respectively.

Author details

Ashraf Alqaqa

Address all correspondence to: ayqs@yahoo.com

Tennova Healthcare, Tennessee, USA

References

[1] Friedman-Kien, A., et al. Kaposis sarcoma and Pneumocystis pneumonia among homosexual men—New York City and California. *MMWR. Morbidity and Mortality Weekly Report*, 1981. **30**(25): 305–308.

[2] Barre-Sinoussi, F., et al. Isolation of T-lymphotropic retrovirus from a patient at risk for acquired immune deficiency syndrome (AIDS). *Revista de investigación clínica*, 2004. **56**(2): 126–129.

[3] Organization, W.H. *Unaids report on the global aids epidemic*. Geneva: UNAIDS and World Health Organization, 2010.

[4] Bayley, A. Surgical pathology of HIV infection: lessons from Africa. *British Journal of Surgery*, 1990. **77**(8): 863–868.

[5] Joshi, V.V., et al. Arteriopathy in children with acquired immune deficiency syndrome. *Fetal and Pediatric Pathology*, 1987. **7**(3): 261–275.

[6] Nair, R., et al. Arterial aneurysms in patients infected with human immunodeficiency virus: a distinct clinicopathology entity? *Journal of Vascular Surgery*, 1999. **29**(4): 600–607.

[7] Chetty, R. Vasculitides associated with HIV infection. *Journal of Clinical Pathology*, 2001. **54**(4): 275–278.

[8] Botes, K., and Van Marle, J. Surgical intervention for HIV related vascular disease. *European Journal of Vascular and Endovascular Surgery*, 2007. **34**(4): 390–396.

[9] Chetty, R., Batitang, S., and Nair, R. Large artery vasculopathy in HIV-positive patients: another vasculitic enigma. *Human Pathology*, 2000. **31**(3): 374–379.

[10] Nair, R., et al. Occlusive arterial disease in HIV-infected patients: a preliminary report. *European Journal of Vascular and Endovascular Surgery*, 2000a. **20**(4): 353–357.

[11] Nair, R., et al. Clinical profile of HIV-related aneurysms. *European Journal of Vascular and Endovascular Surgery*, 2000b. **20**(3): 235–240.

[12] Mulaudzi, T. HIV-associated vasculopathy. *Continuing Medical Education*, 2009. **27**(7): 320–322.

[13] Bulsara, K.R., Raja, A., and Owen, J. HIV and cerebral aneurysms. *Neurosurgical Review*, 2005. **28**(2): 92–95.

[14] Tipping, B., et al. Stroke caused by human immunodeficiency virus–associated intracranial large-vessel aneurysmal vasculopathy. *Archives of Neurology*, 2006. **63**(11): 1640–1642.

[15] Kossorotoff, M., et al. Cerebral vasculopathy with aneurysm formation in HIV-infected young adults. *Neurology*, 2006. **66**(7): 1121–1122.

[16] Periard, D., Cavassini, M., Taffé, P., Chevalley, M., Senn, L., Chapuis-Taillard, C., de Vallière, S., Hayoz, D., Tarr, P.E., Swiss HIV Cohort Study. High prevalence of peripheral arterial disease in HIV-infected persons. *Clinical Infectious Diseases*, 2008. **46**(5): 761–767.

[17] Benjamin, L.A., Bryer, A., Emsley, H.C., Khoo, S., Solomon, T., Connor, M.D. HIV infection and stroke: current perspectives and future directions. *The Lancet Neurology*, 2012. **11**(10): 878–890.

[18] Woolgar, J., et al. Colour doppler and grey scale ultrasound features of HIV-related vascular aneurysms. *The British Journal of Radiology*, 2002. **75**(899): 884–888.

[19] Committee, W., Cardio-and cerebrovascular events in HIV-infected persons. *AIDS*, 2004. **18**(13): 1811–1817.

[20] Law, M., et al. Modelling the 3-year risk of myocardial infarction among participants in the data collection on adverse events of anti-HIV drugs (DAD) study. *HIV Medicine*, 2003. **4**(1): 1–10.

[21] Dubé, M.P., et al. Effects of HIV infection and antiretroviral therapy on the heart and vasculature. *Circulation*, 2008. **118**(2): e36–e40.

[22] Khunnawat, C., et al. Cardiovascular manifestations in human immunodeficiency virus-infected patients. *The American Journal of Cardiology*, 2008. **102**(5): 635–642.

[23] Friis-Moller, N., et al. Class of antiretroviral drugs and the risk of myocardial infarction. *The New England Journal of Medicine*, 2007. **356**(17): 1723–1735.

[24] Mehta, N.J., and Khan, I.A. HIV-associated coronary artery disease. *Angiology*, 2003. **54**(3): 269–275.

[25] Shingadia, D., et al. Takayasu's arteritis in a human immunodeficiency virus—infected adolescent. *Clinical Infectious Diseases*, 1999. **29**(2): 458–459.

[26] Hsue, P.Y., et al. Progression of atherosclerosis as assessed by carotid intima-media thickness in patients with HIV infection. *Circulation*, 2004. **109**(13): 1603–1608.

[27] Calza, L., Manfredi, R., and Chiodo, F. Statins and fibrates for the treatment of hyperlipidaemia in HIV-infected patients receiving HAART. *AIDS*, 2003. **17**(6): 851–859.

[28] Boccara, F., Teiger, E., and Cohen, A. Stent implantation for acute left main coronary artery occlusion in an HIV-infected patient on protease inhibitors. *The Journal of Invasive Cardiology*, 2002. **14**(6): 343–346.

[29] Boccara, F., et al. Clinical characteristics and mid-term prognosis of acute coronary syndrome in HIV-infected patients on antiretroviral therapy. *HIV Medicine*, 2005. **6**(4): 240–244.

[30] Tabib, A., et al. Accelerated coronary atherosclerosis and arteriosclerosis in young human-immunodeficiency-virus-positive patients. *Coronary Artery Disease*, 2000. **11**(1): 41–46.

[31] Rickerts, V., et al. Incidence of myocardial infarctions in HIV-infected patients between 1983 and 1998: the Frankfurt HIV-cohort study. *European Journal of Medical Research*, 2000. **5**(8): 329–333.

[32] Klein, D., et al. Do protease inhibitors increase the risk for coronary heart disease in patients with HIV-1 infection? *Journal of Acquired Immune Deficiency Syndromes (1999)*, 2002. **30**(5): 471–477.

[33] Friis-Moller, N., et al. Combination antiretroviral therapy and the risk of myocardial infarction. *New England Journal of Medicine*, 2003. **349**(21): 1993–2003.

[34] Alqaqa, A., et al. Cardiac sequelae of human immunodeficiency virus disease. *The American Journal of the Medical Sciences*. 2014. **348**(1): 82–86. doi:10.1097/MAJ.0000000000000258. Review.

[35] Hsue, P.Y., et al. Clinical features of acute coronary syndromes in patients with human immunodeficiency virus infection. *Circulation*, 2004. **109**(3): 316–319.

[36] Matetzky, S., et al. Acute myocardial infarction in human immunodeficiency virus–infected patients. *Archives of Internal Medicine*, 2003. **163**(4): 457–460.

[37] Escaut, L., et al. Coronary artery disease in HIV infected patients. *Intensive Care Medicine*, 2003. **29**(6): 969–973.

[38] Boccara, F., et al. Percutaneous coronary intervention in HIV infected patients: immediate results and long term prognosis. *Heart*, 2006. **92**(4): 543–544.

[39] Blyth, D., et al. An experience with cardiopulmonary bypass in HIV-infected patients. *Cardiovascular Journal of South Africa: Official Journal for Southern Africa Cardiac Society [and] South African Society of Cardiac Practitioners*, 2005. **17**(4): 178–185.

[40] Trachiotis, G.D., et al. Cardiac surgery in patients infected with the human immunodeficiency virus. *The Annals of Thoracic Surgery*, 2003. **76**(4): 1114–1118.

[41] Castillo, J.G., et al. Cardiovascular surgery in patients with HIV: epidemiology, current indications, and long-term outcome. *Revista Española de Cardiología (English Edition)*, 2008. **61**(5): 480–486.

[42] Mulaudzi, T., et al. Thrombectomy in HIV related peripheral arterial thrombosis: a preliminary report. *European Journal of Vascular and Endovascular Surgery*, 2005. **30**(1): 102–106.

[43] Boccara, F., et al. Coronary artery bypass graft in HIV-infected patients: a multicenter case control study. *Current HIV Research*, 2008. **6**(1): 59–64.

[44] Sagcan, A., et al. Spontaneous bilateral perirenal hematoma as a complication of polyarteritis nodosa in a patient with human immunodeficiency virus infection. *Rheumatology International*, 2002. **21**(6): 239–242.

[45] Yonou, H., et al. Simultaneous bilateral perirenal hematomas developing spontaneously in a patient with polyarteritis nodosa. *The Journal of Urology*, 1999. **162**(2): 483.

[46] Qaqa, A.Y., et al. Epidemiologic aspects of abnormal ankle brachial index in the HIV infected population. *International Angiology*. 2012. **31**(3): 227–233. Erratum in: *International Angiology*, 2013. **32**(2): 260.

[47] Qaqa, A.Y., et al. The role of postexercise measurements in the diagnosis of peripheral arterial disease in HIV-infected patients. *Angiology*, 2011. **62**(1): 10–14.

Chapter 3

Anti-Retroviral–Based HIV Pre-Exposure Prophylaxis for Women: Recent Advances and Next Steps

Flavia Matovu Kiweewa, Kenneth K. Mugwanya and Francis Kiweewa

Additional information is available at the end of the chapter

http://dx.doi.org/10.5772/67163

Abstract

There is a daunting challenge to prevent human immunodeficiency virus (HIV) acquisition in women at high risk of acquiring HIV. Of the 37 million people globally living with HIV, more than half are women. Women account for nearly 60% of adults with HIV in sub-Saharan Africa, where unprotected heterosexual sex is the primary driver of the epidemic. While male condoms are effective, they are not always used, and this is not something women can control. Women urgently need prevention tools they can decide to use, independent of a husband or partner. Pre-exposure prophylaxis (PrEP), in which HIV-uninfected persons with ongoing HIV risk use antiretroviral (ARV) medications as chemoprophylaxis against sexual HIV acquisition, is a promising new HIV prevention strategy. We review recent advances in the development of new biomedical HIV prevention interventions with a highlight of findings from pivotal clinical trials, as well as a discussion on future generation strategies for women.

Keywords: HIV, women, tenofovir, dapivirine, pre-exposure prophylaxis

1. Introduction

In 2015, 2.1 million people became newly infected with Human Immuno Deficiency Virus (HIV) and 1.1 million died from Acquired Immuno Deficiency Syndrome (AIDS) related illnesses [1]. According to the Joint United Nations Programme on HIV/AIDS (UNAIDS) Global Report, 70 percent of the 37 million people estimated to be living with HIV reside in sub-Saharan Africa [1]. In this setting, where unprotected heterosexual sex is the primary driver of the epidemic, women account for nearly 60 percent of adults with HIV.

While existing HIV-1 prevention interventions including behavior change, use of male and female condoms, treatment of sexually transmitted infections (STIs), male circumcision, and uptake of antiretroviral (ARV) treatment to reduce the infectiousness of persons with HIV-1 have gone a long way in controlling the spread of HIV-1 infection [2–6], HIV-1 rates in young women in resource limited settings remain unacceptably high [1]. This is in part, because many HIV-1 prevention methods require the participation or consent of a male partner. Women urgently need prevention tools they can decide to use, independent of a husband or partner [7]. Developing HIV prevention options that women can use therefore remains a global concern, given the soaring rates of HIV infection among women. Pre-exposure prophylaxis (PrEP), in which HIV uninfected persons with ongoing HIV risk use antiretroviral medications as chemoprophylaxis against sexual HIV acquisition, is a promising new HIV prevention strategy [8–11].

2. HIV prevention biomedical interventions

2.1. Microbicides

2.1.1. CAPRISA 004

Tenofovir gel was the first ARV-based microbicide to be tested in an effectiveness trial. CAPRISA 004 was a phase 2B microbicide study that tested peri-coitally applied 1% TDF vaginal gel among 889 South African women conducted from May 2007 to March 2010. The trial found a 39% (95% CI, 6–60%; p = 0.017) lower HIV infection rate in women using 1% tenofovir gel as compared to the women using placebo gel when used in a coitally dependent regimen [12]. Tenofovir gel was shown to be safe when used up to 12 h before sex and again within 12 h after sex (BAT), for a maximum of two doses in 24 h. The drug was found to be 54% effective among women who were the highest adherers (gel adherence > 80%). Participants who adhered to the dosing regimen in more than 80% of sex acts were the least likely to acquire HIV (54% lower risk of infection).

2.1.2. FACTS 001

FACTS 001 was a phase III safety and effectiveness double-blind, randomised, placebo-controlled trial of pericoital tenofovir 1% gel for HIV prevention in 18–30 year Women at nine sites in South Africa [17]. The study evaluated the safety and effectiveness of pericoital TFV 1% gel when using the BAT-24 regimen (before and after sex; no more than 2 doses in 24 h) among women at nine sites in South Africa. A total of 2059 women were randomized to tenofovir 1% gel or to placebo and instructed women to apply the gel 12 h before and within 12 h after sex, the same schedule used in CAPRISA 004. The study was conducted between Oct 2011 and Aug 2014. In 3036 person-years of observation accrued, 123 HIV infections occurred (HIV incidence: 4.0/100 women years); 61 in the TFV arm and 62 in the placebo group (incidence rate ratio [IRR], 1.0; 95% CI: 0.7–1.4). In a nested case-cohort sub-study (n = 214) that examined TFV drug levels in quarterly cervicovaginal lavage (CVL) samples in HIV seroconverters vs controls, high TFV in CVL was significantly associated with a reduction in HIV acquisition (HR, 0.52; 95% CI, 0.27–0.99; p = 0.04).

Considering all adherence data, the FACTS 001 team calculated that women used gel for an average of 50–60% of sex acts. Majority of participants were not able to achieve sufficiently high levels of gel coverage required for protection which underscores the need for a range of HIV prevention options for young women which may be easier to integrate into their lives.

2.2. Oral PrEP

2.2.1. Partner's PrEP

The Partners PrEP Study was a three-arm phase III, randomized, double-blind, placebo-controlled, 3-arm trial of daily oral TDF & FTC/TDF PrEP for the prevention of HIV acquisition by HIV seronegative partner in heterosexual HIV serodiscordant partnerships. It was one of the two land marker studies that provided evidence to support US Food and Drug Administration approval for FTC-TDF PrEP. The study demonstrated PrEP HIV protective effectiveness against HIV infection of 67% (95% CI 44–81%, p < 0.0001) for TDF and 75% (95% CI 55–87%, p < 0.0001) for FTC/TDF [13] compared to person receiving placebo. The HIV protection effects of TDF and FTC/TDF were in women and men. For TDF, efficacy among women was 71% and was 63% among men; for FTC/TDF, efficacy was 66% in women and 84% in men—all were statistically significant. In a follow-on open-label demonstration project of integrated delivery of ART and PrEP for prevention in HIV sero-discordant couples, the investigators observed virtual elimination of incident HIV [13].

2.2.2. FEM-PrEP Study

The FEM-PrEP Study was a phase 3, randomized, placebo-controlled, trial that assessed of the effectiveness of daily oral FTC/TDF for HIV prevention among HIV-uninfected women 18–35 years in Kenya, South Africa and Tanzania [14]. The trial was stopped early by Independent Data Monitoring Committee due to futility at the time of study stop. No significant safety concerns were noted. Adherence by self-report and pill counts was high, but plasma drug levels revealed that only 15–26% of samples from seroconverters had TDF detected and only 26–38% of non-seroconverting controls. Thus, the investigators concluded that PrEP adherence was too low to assess PrEP's HIV protection. Less than 40% of the HIV-uninfected women in the TDF–FTC group had evidence of recent pill use at visits that were matched to the HIV-infection window for women with seroconversion.

2.2.3. TDF2 study

The TDF2 study was a phase 2B study that assessed the safety, adherence and efficacy of daily oral FTC/TDF in 1200 (45.7% women) HIV-uninfected heterosexual male and female participants aged 18–39 years conducted in Botswana [15]. After a 1563 person-years of observation (median, 1.1 years; maximum, 3.7 years), FTC/TDF PrEP resulted in a 62.6% reduction in HIV acquisition for participants assigned to FTC/TDF compared to placebo (HR, 0.37; CI, 21.5–83.4, p = 0.013). As treated analysis provided protective efficacy of 77.9% (95% CI, 41.2–93.6; p = 0.01) for FTC/TDF versus placebo, overall, and 75.4% (23.7, 94.4; p = 0.02) for women. No significant safety concerns were noted, though participants randomized to the FTC/TDF arm did experience more nausea, vomiting and dizziness than those randomized to placebo.

2.2.4. MTN-003/Vaginal and Oral Interventions to Control the Epidemic (VOICE)

Was a phase 2B safety and effectiveness study of tenofovir 1% gel, tenofovir disoproxil fumarate tablet and emtricitabine/tenofovir disoproxil fumarate tablet for the prevention of HIV infection in women [16]. The primary aim of the VOICE trial was to estimate the safety and effectiveness of daily treatment with vaginal TFV gel, as compared with placebo gel, and of oral TDF and oral TDF-FTC, as compared with oral placebo, in preventing sexually acquired HIV-1 infection in women.

A total of 5029 were enrolled in the study were followed up monthly and assessed for HIV seroconversion. A total of 312 HIV-1 infections occurred; the incidence of HIV-1 infection was 5.7 per 100 person-years. In the modified intention-to-treat analysis, the effectiveness was −49.0% with TDF (hazard ratio for infection, 1.49; 95% confidence interval [CI], 0.97–2.29), −4.4% with TDF-FTC (hazard ratio, 1.04; 95% CI, 0.73–1.49), and 14.5% with TFV gel (hazard ratio, 0.85; 95% CI, 0.61–1.21). Adherence to study product among those in the active arms was generally very low. TFV was detectable in 30%, 29%, and 25% of random plasma samples from participants in the TDF, TDF-FTC, and TFV gel arms of the study, and an inverse correlation was demonstrable between detection of TFV in plasma and characteristics predictive of HIV-1 acquisition.

2.2.5. Partner's demonstration project

OLE projects have been called for as part of the pathway to scale-up of PrEP. Previous studies like the Partner's PrEP that assessed effectiveness of oral truvada and tenofovir for HIV prevention among sero-discordant couples in Kenya and Uganda have shown that when participants are given the active product through open-label access projects, even those with previous poor adherence during the clinical trial are now more likely to use product when they know they are now using the active product [13]. From a protection level of about 73% in the partner's PrEP, researchers have reported substantially reduced HIV risk of up to 95% when used with high adherence [17], **Figure 1**.

2.3. Vaginal rings

2.3.1. MTN-020— A Study to Prevent HIV Infection with a Ring with Extended ring (ASPIRE)

Intravaginal rings offer a strategy to deliver antiretroviral PrEP medications with lesser opportunities for adherence challenges than for daily oral pills or vaginal gels [18]. ASPIRE was a phase III study conducted among 2629 sexually active HIV-negative women ages 18–45 at 15 clinical research sites in Malawi, Uganda, South Africa and Zimbabwe to determine whether a vaginal ring containing the ARV drug dapivirine is a safe and effective method for protecting against the sexual transmission of HIV when used by women for a month at a time. The study found HIV risk was reduced by 27% overall—for women group assigned to use the dapivirine ring compared placebo ring group—and 37% in a planned second analysis that excluded data from two sites with less than ideal retention and adherence. Notably high protection (56%) was observed in women >21 years, who also appeared to use the ring most consistently, **Figure 2** [10].

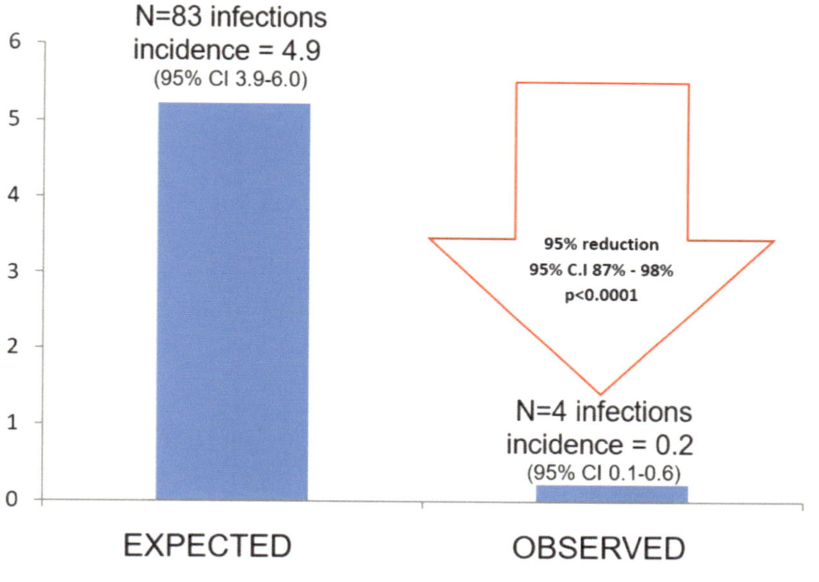

Figure 1. HIV incidence in Partner's PrEP demonstration project [17].

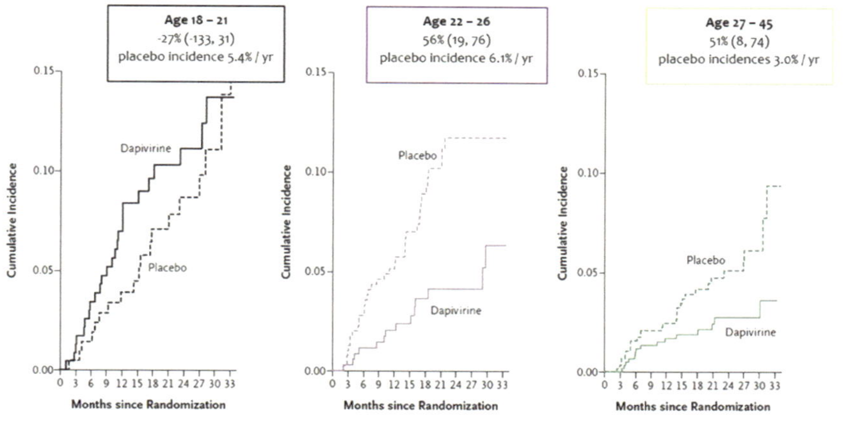

Figure 2. Age and HIV-1 protection in ASPIRE [10].

A summary of the outcomes of recent HIV prevention trials among women is provided in **Table 1**.

Study	Study population	Sample size	Results
CAPRISA 004 *South Africa* (Tenofovir Gel)	Women	889	39% [CI = 6–60] effectiveness of coitally-dependent vaginal TFV gel
iPrEx *Brazil, Ecuador, Peru, South Africa, Thailand, US* (Oral Truvada)	Gay men, other MSM, transgender women	2499	44% [CI = 15–63] effectiveness of daily oral FTC/TDF
TDF2 Study *Botswana* (Oral Tenofovir)	Men and women	1200	62% [CI = 22–83] effectiveness of daily oral FTC/TDF
Partners PrEP Study *Kenya, Uganda* (Oral Truvada/Tenofovir)	Serodiscordant couples	4758	67% [CI = 44–81] efficacy daily oral TDF 75% [CI = 55–87] efficacy daily oral FTC/TDF
FEM-PrEP *Kenya, S Africa, Tanzania* (Oral Truvada)	Women	1950	Futility of daily oral FTC/TDF 6% [CI = −52 to 41]
ASPIRE *Uganda, Malawi, South Africa, Zimbabwe*	Women	2629	27% [CI= 1–46] effectiveness of dapivirine vaginal ring

Table 1. Outcomes of recent HIV prevention trials involving women.

2.3.2. MTN-025—HIV open-label prevention extension (HOPE)

HOPE is an open-label study of vaginal ring for preventing HIV among former ASPIRE participants. Women who took part in ASPIRE, a trial that found a vaginal ring containing an antiretroviral (ARV) drug called dapivirine was safe and helped protect against HIV, are now being offered the opportunity to use the ring as part of a new study called HOPE. HOPE builds on the results of ASPIRE by gathering additional information on the ring's safety, how women use the ring knowing that it can help reduce their risk of HIV and the relationship between adherence and HIV protection. Women who participated in a similar study called the RING study by the international partnership for microbicides (IPM) are being followed up under the dapivirine ring extended access and monitoring (DREAM OLE) protocol.

2.4. Discussion

High HIV incidence among young women in Africa [1] highlights the need for female-controlled HIV prevention. Social, structural and economic disparities perpetuate vulnerabilities of women. The lower social and economic power of women makes it difficult for them to negotiate safe sex [18]. In stable partnerships, condom use is low, and women are often unaware of their partner's HIV status [19]. Therefore, a need exists for HIV prevention methods that

http://dx.doi.org/10.5772/67163

women can initiate themselves. Scaling up of proven biomedical technologies for women at high risk is therefore a high priority. Daily oral tenofovir-based PrEP, dapivirine vaginal ring and antiretroviral treatment as prevention are some of the promising biomedical technologies for prevention options for women.

Multiple studies of PrEP have shown that oral ARVs, when used consistently, reduce the risk of HIV infection in people who are at high risk by up to 92% including among women [5]. Currently, FTC-TDF is the medication with a label indication as PrEP against HIV acquisition recommended by the World Health Organization (WHO) and the United States Centers of Diseases Control and Prevention [20, 21]. Consequently, recent landmark approvals in sub-Saharan Africa, including South Africa [22] and Kenya [23], and commitment from large-scale funding partners (including PEPFAR) are leading to accelerated roll-out of TDF-based PrEP for high-risk populations. TDF alone or TDF with lamivudine are other as an alternative to suggested by WHO [24]. Importantly, other new oral PrEP drugs (e.g. maraviroc) are currently being evaluated [25]. Although some PrEP trials in African women did not show effectiveness against HIV [14, 16, 26], follow-on analyses from those two studies have consistently provided strong evidence of very low adherence to PrEP in those studies [16, 27].

Prevention technologies such as vaginal ring containing ARV provide tremendous promise for the HIV prevention field as they provide HIV prevention options that fit in women's lives. The recent demonstration of moderate HIV protection conferred by monthly vaginal ring containing medication dapivirine is a step in right direction. An important feature of the dapivirine ring is its high level of safety [28]. This excellent safety profile also suggests that minimal medical monitoring would be needed, potentially making it both a practical and cost-effective option in under-resourced settings. The next step is to ensure that the vaginal ring is safe for all women at risk of HIV acquisition including pregnant and breastfeeding women.

For HIV uninfected women in known serodiscorant partnership, initiation and sustained use of ART by their infected male patterns are another highly effective prevention options for couples [5]. Women who want to conceive or with HIV positive partners who have not yet initiated ART, PrEP as bridge to ART prevention strategy is an attractive and highly effective HIV option. In PrEP as a bridge to ART strategy, PrEP is offered to HIV-uninfected person as a 'bridge' to ART in the discordant partnership—that is, until ART initiation by the HIV-infected partner and for the first 6 months after ART is started or viral suppression. This strategy demonstrated nearly elimination of HIV transmission within serodiscordant couples in Uganda and Kenya [29].

A robust pipeline of new PrEP drugs and formulations is not only important for advancing demonstrated success of products but also for addressing limitations of current biomedical technologies with the ultimate goal of prevention options that fit women's needs to ensure they will be used at scale. The current pipeline of ARV-based prevention products includes oral pills (miravorac), vaginal rings (tenofovir), vaginal and rectal gels, vaginal films, long-acting injectable ARVs (rilpivirine, cabotegravir) and multipurpose technologies that could combine ARV to reduce women's risk of HIV and STIs while providing effective contraception.

3. Summary

Oral PrEP trials have demonstrated a decrease in HIV infection rates of between 44 and 77%. But it is now proven that with good adherence, Truvada, a once-a-day pill can reduce HIV infection rates by at least 92%. Because of high level of effectiveness, oral PrEP has been licensed for high-risk populations in the US, Canada, Kenya and South Africa. Efforts to have the dapivirine vaginal ring licensed for HIV prevention among women are currently underway. The process is an important one that takes time. It's anticipated that regulatory approvals could be received by 2018 in some countries in Africa. Results of the ASPIRE and RING studies are a boost to efforts focused on developing and evaluating next generation products, such a 3-month ring (just four rings would provide a woman a full year of protection), and combination rings that can provide protection against HIV, other STIs and unintended pregnancy. A vaginal ring could offer an important option as part of combination strategies or as a stand-alone method for women unable or not willing to use other strategies like medical male circumcision, condoms and oral PrEP.

Author details

Flavia Matovu Kiweewa[1,2,*], Kenneth K. Mugwanya[1,3] and Francis Kiweewa[1,4]

*Address all correspondence to: fmatovu@mujhu.org

1 Makerere University School of Public Health, Makerere University College of Health Sciences, Kampala, Uganda

2 University of Witwatersrand, Johannesburg, South Africa

3 University of Washington, Seattle, United States

4 Makerere University-Walter Reed Project, Kampala, Uganda

References

[1] UNAIDS. Report on the global AIDS epidemic 2015.

[2] Seidman D, Weber S, Aaron E, Cohan D, Grant R. The FACTS about women and pre-exposure prophylaxis. The Lancet HIV. 2015;2(6):e228.

[3] Gray RH, Kigozi G, Serwadda D, Makumbi F, Watya S, Nalugoda F, et al. Male circumcision for HIV prevention in men in Rakai, Uganda: a randomised trial. The Lancet. 2007;369(9562):657–66.

[4] Weiss HA, Halperin D, Bailey RC, Hayes RJ, Schmid G, Hankins CA. Male circumcision for HIV prevention: from evidence to action? AIDS. 2008;22(5):567–74.

[5] Cohen MS, McCauley M, Gamble TR. HIV treatment as prevention and HPTN 052. Current Opinion in HIV and AIDS. 2012;7(2):99.

[6] Patterson TL, Shaw WS, Semple SJ. Reducing the sexual risk behaviors of HIV+ individuals: outcome of a randomized controlled trial. Annals of Behavioral Medicine. 2003;25(2):137–45.

[7] Wawer MJ, Sewankambo NK, Serwadda D, Quinn TC, Kiwanuka N, Li C, et al. Control of sexually transmitted diseases for AIDS prevention in Uganda: a randomised community trial. The Lancet. 1999;353(9152):525–35.

[8] Elias CJ, Coggins C. Female-controlled methods to prevent sexual transmission of HIV. AIDS (London, England). 1996;10:S43–51.

[9] Jiang J, Yang X, Ye L, Zhou B, Ning C, Huang J, et al. Pre-exposure prophylaxis for the prevention of HIV infection in high risk populations: a meta-analysis of randomized controlled trials. PLoS One. 2014;9(2):e87674.

[10] Baeten JM, Grant R. Use of antiretrovirals for HIV prevention: what do we know and what don't we know? Current HIV/AIDS Reports. 2013;10(2):142–51.

[11] Control CfD, Prevention. Update to Interim Guidance for Preexposure Prophylaxis (PrEP) for the Prevention of HIV Infection: PrEP for injecting drug users. MMWR Morbidity and Mortality Weekly Report. 2013;62(23):463.

[12] Karim QA, Karim SSA, Frohlich JA, Grobler AC, Baxter C, Mansoor LE, et al. Effectiveness and safety of tenofovir gel, an antiretroviral microbicide, for the prevention of HIV infection in women. Science. 2010;329(5996):1168–74.

[13] Baeten JM, Heffron R, Kidoguchi L, Mugo NR, Katabira E, Bukusi EA, et al. Integrated delivery of antiretroviral treatment and pre-exposure prophylaxis to HIV-1–serodiscordant couples: a prospective implementation study in Kenya and Uganda. PLoS Medicine. 2016;13(8):e1002099.

[14] Van Damme L, Corneli A, Ahmed K, Agot K, Lombaard J, Kapiga S, et al. Preexposure prophylaxis for HIV infection among African women. New England Journal of Medicine. 2012;367(5):411–22.

[15] Thigpen MC, Kebaabetswe PM, Paxton LA, Smith DK, Rose CE, Segolodi TM, et al. Antiretroviral preexposure prophylaxis for heterosexual HIV transmission in Botswana. New England Journal of Medicine. 2012;367(5):423–34.

[16] Marrazzo JM, Ramjee G, Richardson BA, Gomez K, Mgodi N, Nair G, et al. Tenofovir-based preexposure prophylaxis for HIV infection among African women. New England Journal of Medicine. 2015;372(6):509–18.

[17] Baeten J, Heffron R, Kidoguchi L, Mugo N, Bukusi E, Katabira E, editors. Near elimination of HIV transmission in a demonstration project of PrEP and ART. Conference on Retroviruses and Opportunistic Infections (CROI); 2015.

[18] Langen TT. Gender power imbalance on women\'s capacity to negotiate self-protection against HIV/AIDS in Botswana and South Africa. African Health Sciences. 2005;5(3):188–97.

[19] Wagner GJ, Holloway I, Ghosh-Dastidar B, Ryan G, Kityo C, Mugyenyi P. Factors associated with condom use among HIV clients in stable relationships with partners at varying risk for HIV in Uganda. AIDS and Behavior. 2010;14(5):1055–65.

[20] Centers for Disease Control and Prevenion. Preexposure prophylaxis for the prevention of HIV infection in the United States-2014: A clinical practice guideline. [Accessed on February 9, 2017];2014 :1–67. http://www.cdc.gov/hiv/pdf/prepguidelines2014.pdf.

[21] World Health Organization. Guideline on when to start antiretroviral therapy and on pre-exposure prophylaxis for HIV. http://apps.who.int/iris/bitstream/10665/186275/1/9789241509565_eng.pdf. Accessed May 10, 2016.

[22] Bekker L-G, Rebe K, Venter F, Maartens G, Moorhouse M, Conradie F, et al. Southern African guidelines on the safe use of pre-exposure prophylaxis in persons at risk of acquiring HIV-1 infection. Southern African Journal of HIV Medicine. 2016;17(1):1–11.

[23] http://emtct-iatt.org/wp-content/uploads/2016/09/Guidelines-on-Use-of-Antiretroviral-Drugs-for-Treating-and-Preventing-HI....pdf Guidelines on Use of Antiretroviral Drugs for Treating and Preventing HIV Infection in Kenya 2016 Edition Accessed October 2016.

[24] World Health Organization. Consolidated guidelines on the use of antiretroviral drugs for treating and preventing HIV infection—recommendations for a public health approach, second edition, 2016. Geneva, Switzerland: World Health Organization, 2016. http://www.who.int/hiv/pub/arv/arv-2016/en/.

[25] Abraham BK, Gulick R. Next generation oral PrEP: beyond tenofovir. Current Opinion in HIV and AIDS. 2012;7(6):600.

[26] Rees H, Delany-Moretlwe S, Lombard C, editors. FACTS 001: a multi-centred phase III randomised, double-blind, placebo-controlled tiral of periocoital tenofovir 1% gel for HIV prevention in Women. Conference on Retroviruses and Opportunistic Infections; 2015.

[27] Corneli AL, Deese J, Wang M, Taylor D, Ahmed K, Agot K, et al. FEM-PrEP: adherence patterns and factors associated with adherence to a daily oral study product for pre-exposure prophylaxis. JAIDS Journal of Acquired Immune Deficiency Syndromes. 2014;66(3):324–31.

[28] Baeten, Jared M., et al. "Antiretroviral prophylaxis for HIV prevention in heterosexual men and women." *New England Journal of Medicine* 367.5 (2012): 399-410.

[29] Heffron R, Pintye J, Matthews LT, Weber S, Mugo N. PrEP as peri-conception HIV prevention for women and men. Current HIV/AIDS Reports. 2016;13:131–9.

Section 2

Social and Economic Aspects

Chapter 4

Three Decades of HIV/AIDS Pandemic: Challenges Faced by Orphans in Tembisa, South Africa

Pius Tangwe Tanga, Princess Khumalo and
Priscilla Gutura

Additional information is available at the end of the chapter

http://dx.doi.org/10.5772/66652

Abstract

This paper was extracted from a broader study conducted on the effectiveness of social support mechanisms provided to human immunodeficiency virus/acquired immunodeficiency syndrome (HIV/AIDS) orphans in Tembisa, Gauteng Province. Using a qualitative research design, an interview guide was designed for in-depth interviews, which were conducted with 12 HIV- and AIDS-affected and -infected orphans. In addition, a focus group discussion was run with 13 children's caregivers and two social workers were interviewed as key informants. Nevertheless, this paper discusses the challenges faced by orphans of HIV and AIDS. Maslow's hierarchy of needs was used as the theoretical framework of the study. The findings indicate that the death of a parent signifies the disruption of the basic pattern of a child's life living in the urban area where the role of extended families does not exist as compared to rural areas where a child belongs to the whole village. There are challenges that are impacting on the daily lives of the HIV/AIDS-affected and -infected orphans. Notably, the participants' narratives suggested that there were challenges in terms of health, shelter, education and food. It is concluded therefore that the war against the impacts of HIV and AIDS is still far from being achieved.

Keywords: HIV and AIDS, social support, challenges, orphans, caregivers, social workers

1. Introduction

Human immunodeficiency virus (HIV) and acquired immunodeficiency syndrome (AIDS) is one of the major public health challenges and it is a pandemic worldwide [1]. Statistics released by Statistics South Africa showed that the population of the country was estimated at 54.96 million by mid-2015 with approximately 48% being male and 52% female [2]. Furthermore,

Statistics SA showed that the estimated overall HIV prevalence rate is approximately 11.2% of the total South African population. The total number of people living with HIV is estimated at approximately 6.19 million in 2015. For adults aged 15–49 years, an estimated 16.6% of the population is HIV positive [2].

Further, HIV/AIDS has increased the number of orphans enormously to the extent that the United Nations in 2000 defines an orphan as a child who has lost one parent. This is because, when the first parent is killed by the disease, the next one follows within a short period of time. The death of both parents leads the child to be called a double orphan [3]. However, in most African nations, the fact of the matter is that the burden of parental death from AIDS is the greatest with 12.3 million children under the age of 15 having lost one or both parents to AIDS [4]. There is an estimation that 12 million children aged 17 and younger in the sub-Saharan Africa have lost one or both parents mainly due to HIV/AIDS [5]. This sordid truth is not far-fetched even in the Southern African region. Then, it was concluded that these children are often left in the care of caregivers who have limited resources and abilities to care and provide for their psychosocial needs [6].

The General Household Survey in 2007 identified approximately 3.7 million orphans (children without both parents) living in South Africa. This survey also indicated that the number of children who had lost both parents had increased over the previous 5 years (2002–2006) and of further interest was that during 2006, 77% of all orphans were of school-going age—7 years and above.

Substantially, there are international articles that place primary responsibility of the welfare of children on parents or guardians and extended families. These are the Convention of the Rights of the Child (CRC) (Article 5) and the African Charter on the Rights and Welfare of the Child (AC) (Articles 9 (3) and 18). However, the African norms and values just like the aforementioned articles also articulate such child-welfare values. Even Kawewe [6] argues that in many African traditions the extended family is part and parcel of child rearing with the villagers and community members playing a role as the child is viewed as belonging to everyone. He further concludes that the AIDS pandemic defies the concept of the analogy 'it takes a village to raise a child' as many communities can no longer cope with those in need of care. As a result, children are left without caregivers. Some are left in alternative care such as adoption, non-relative care or institutionalization.

South Africa is a signatory to the Declaration of Commitment of the United Nations General Assembly Special Session on Children held in 2002 (UNGASS). One of the articles of the Declaration states that

> By 2003 develop, and by 2005 implement national policies and strategies to:
>
> Build and strengthen governmental family and community capacities to provide supportive environments for orphans and boys and girls infected and affected by HIV and tAIDS including by providing appropriate counselling and psycho-social support, ensuring their enrolment in school and access to shelter, good nutrition, health and social services on an equal basis with other children, to protect orphans and vulnerable children from all forms of abuse, violence, exploitation, discrimination, trafficking and loss of inheritance. (Article 65)

In the past few years of the post-apartheid regime, profound political and social changes have been seen in South Africa, with the government taking the lead in introducing significant social welfare policy changes [7]. Major objectives of social welfare policies in South Africa are alleviating poverty and enabling the previously disadvantaged communities to have access to basic social services [8]. The social security system (mainly social grants) is the government's chief initiative in tackling poverty and inequality through which, according to [9], it has over 16 million beneficiaries accessing the social grants provided for by the government. Among these grants is a grant for children known as the Foster Care Grant.

The Foster Care Grant is also used to provide support for children orphaned by HIV and AIDS; it is orphans who have lost both parents who are the most likely to be receiving the grant, providing that children remain in the care of foster parents [10]. Partially reflecting the effects of a deepening HIV and AIDS pandemic, since 10 years ago, when HIV-related orphaning rates started rising rapidly, the use of the Foster Care Grant changed. The number of Foster Care Grant beneficiaries rose from 43,000 in 1997 to 300,000 in 2006 [11]. As of 30 April 2016, approximately 545,000 children were receiving the Foster Care Grant [9].

The Sowetan reported that the Social Development Minister Bathabile Dlamini, in Gugulethu, had highlighted that caregivers were reported to be misusing social grants [12]. According to the government, these social assistance grants are to assist caregivers to give orphans (in this case, HIV and AIDS orphans) a better life, a chance to be respectable members of the community and reduce poverty. However, a number of studies carried out so far have indicated that child poverty is still exceedingly high [13, 14]. According to UNICEF's report on the level of child poverty, it was clearly indicated that poverty was deepening in various parts of South Africa [4]. It was further argued that poverty and unemployment are key concerns that impact on a family's capacity to care for their children [7]. They also noted that previous inequalities in education, health care and basic infrastructure have also contributed to the backlog in present services [7]. The vulnerability of children, especially those living in poor areas, is compounded by HIV and AIDS.

A number of researchers [15, 16] have indicated that the HIV and AIDS pandemic is one of the greatest threats to the realization of child rights in South Africa and sub-Saharan Africa. Research by the Children's Institute demonstrates some of the multiple vulnerabilities faced by children before the death of caregivers [17]. Children often take on the responsibility of caring for sick adults and are unable to attend school or study because of the difficulties at home. In short, children's experiences of orphanhood and its compounded vulnerabilities begin long before the death of a significant adult. It is not surprising that many of the subsequent experiences of children who have been orphaned are poverty-related—such as an inability to afford school fees and school uniforms, prolonged experiences of hunger, inadequate housing and poor access to water [17]. On the other hand, Meintjes and Hall [18] reported that although the government and civil society have expressed concern about the growing number of children living in child-headed households, there is little evidence to support this fear.

The Department of Social Development provides care and support to orphans and vulnerable children and their caregivers and these include child-care forums, community-based drop-ins, home-based care centres, early childhood development programmes, among others. For the purpose of this study, support mechanisms refer to all social support given to HIV and AIDS orphans in Tembisa Child and Family Welfare Society Organization. This assistance might be from social workers, care workers or givers and other members of society, offering support to orphans affected and infected with HIV and AIDS. The need for continuing social welfare policy reform processes and providing support mechanisms for responding to orphans and vulnerable children in South Africa is critical for policymakers. This research therefore evaluated the social support provided to HIV and AIDS orphans in Tembisa, Gauteng. A huge emphasis is placed on the challenges faced. The study focused more on the challenges faced by female caregivers as they form the bulk of Tembisa Child and Family Welfare Society's caseloads and the HIV and AIDS orphans in their care.

2. The research problem

The AIDS epidemic has affected many children in South Africa leaving them either affected or infected [19]. These children are left behind with the greatest challenge of all which is figuring out how to survive, they are left with responsibilities way beyond their capacities, and they lack financial, emotional, physical, mental and material support to care for themselves. In addition, they are left under the care of people who are financially, emotionally, physically or mentally incapable to care for them [20]. The government has put forward means to assist these children to cope with the difficulties of life, but regardless of these there is still a need to determine how effective the measures put forward are assisting.

The majority of orphans and vulnerable children in South Africa are left in the care of old and weak women or sickly caregivers. The government has made recommendable success in combating abject poverty and hunger through social assistance programme [21]. Even after such measures, issues such as fraud still hover around and most caregivers and orphans are still battling with meeting challenges of day-to-day living. However, [21] continues to argue that the high prevalence of HIV and AIDS among caregivers has worsened the challenges of child poverty. The government in 2005 enacted the Children's Act 38 of 2005 which provided under Section 155 and 156 for the orphans of whatever nature to be associated with Foster Care Grants. The grant was to assist foster parents put the orphaned children through school, clothe them and shelter them. Due to the backlogs in many organizations assisting with the application of these grants and the misuse of such grants by some foster parents, the survival of HIV and AIDS orphans is still a struggle far from being won. The previous inequalities in education, health care and basic infrastructure have highly contributed in caregivers being unable to care for orphans and orphaned children [21].

3. Theoretical framework

This study is anchored on Maslow's theory of human needs [22]. Maslow's theory of human needs depicts the hierarchy in a manner where needs in the lower level should be met before an individual can progress and satisfy the needs in the next level. This theory has five levels of needs, the lowest being the most basic need that a body cannot survive without and the top of the pyramid the least basic human need [23]. The lowest level of the pyramid is physiological needs, safety and security needs, love and belonging needs; at the top of the pyramid are esteem needs and self-actualization. Once a need is satisfied an individual will be able to go to the next need [24].

This theory is relevant in this study as HIV/AIDS orphans have needs that should be met in order to fulfil their responsibilities. Orphans are driven by several factors to strive to satisfy the bottom need, and then move on up the hierarchy. Therefore, through understanding their challenges as AIDS orphans, ways of motivating them to fulfil their lives can be developed and implemented.

4. Research area and methodology

Data presented in this paper were collected from Tembisa and the participants included HIV/AIDS orphans and their caregivers and social workers. The purpose was to get views from both the orphans themselves and the people who cared for these orphans. It is believed that once the researcher has developed an understanding of the rationale behind the choice of engaging in any form of research (either qualitative or quantitative), he designs the study [25]. Therefore, a qualitative research design was selected for this study. The goal of this method was to learn about the phenomenon and get in-depth information and feelings of the participants.

The study was conducted in Tembisa Township in the East Rand of the Gauteng province in South Africa. The township is just a few kilometres outside the Kempton Park and the second largest township in Gauteng after Soweto. Its population is estimated to be a little over 500,000. The township came about during the apartheid era as a beacon of hope to the black families who were evicted from their homes. Many people live in poverty and in shacks or the recently built houses from the government (Reconstruction and Development Programme). Tembisa Child and Family Welfare Society provides social services to the township, especially for HIV/AIDS orphans and their caregivers.

This study was only limited to HIV and AIDS orphans being serviced by Tembisa Child and Family Welfare Society and also residing there. The study also targeted the caregivers of the orphans and the social workers who were servicing them. Therefore, this research made use of 13 caregivers, two social workers and 12 orphans. For the purpose of this study, the non-probability procedure in the form of purposive sampling was utilized to select the sample. The orphans were selected purposefully from the database of HIV and AIDS orphans receiving services from Tembisa Child and Family Welfare Society. The samples were drawn from the caseloads of social workers.

The study used semi-structured interviews with the aid of interview guides. The interview guide consisted of non-directive unstructured questions which were written in English, but the interviews were conducted in both English and Zulu. The questions on the research guide were meant to guide the researcher to keep to the objectives of the study. The interviews conducted were recorded with an audio recorder to make it easy to capture all the data and also to avoid misquoting the participants.

Focus groups were also used as a method of collecting data and they targeted care givers. Focus groups are a means of understanding how people feel or think about an issue [26] and can help understand how people feel about the issue being studied. Participants in the focus groups were allowed to share their perceptions, points of views, experiences and wishes without any pressure. An environment that is tolerant and non-threatening to all participants was created. Once the research reached a point of saturation [27], the data collection process was concluded.

Qualitative data analysis was used. Data analysis was explained as the process of bringing order, structure and meaning to a mass of data collected [26]. Qualitative data analysis according to Ref. [26] is a search for general statements about relationships in different categories of data. The researchers went through the transcripts of the collected data with the use of a translator. Data analysis was done through the process of thematic analysis. Through reading the transcripts, the researcher came up with the underlying meanings of the information gathered. This process was repeated until a list of topics was acquired. Topics were then clustered together into baskets and were labelled as 'major topics', 'unique topics' and 'leftovers'. Data were then categorized into themes after finding the most descriptive wording for the topics [26].

In line with the ethical requirements of research, the researchers consulted with relevant authorities to gain access to research components. In order to gain access to the participants, the researchers firstly gained permission from the university in the form of an ethical clearance certificate. Other ethical procedures, including informed consent, anonymity and confidentiality, as well as participant debriefing were put into place during and after data collection. Potential respondents were verbally informed at the start of the study that their participation was completely voluntary and verbal consent of their participation was obtained. Caregivers provided verbal consent for themselves and their children. The children themselves gave consent for their participation and child-friendly language was used.

5. Results

This section provides the findings of the study, according to the themes that emerged. Firstly, the biographical information of the participants is laid out. Thereafter, the challenges faced by orphans, caregivers and social workers are presented.

5.1. Biographical characteristics of participants

Interviews were held with 12 orphans within the age range of 10–18 (both affected and/infected with HIV and AIDS). In terms of gender, these children were proportionately selected, that is, they consisted of six males and six females. A total number of eight children interviewed were both affected and infected with HIV and AIDS and four indicated that they were affected only. Seven of the orphans were maternal orphans with unknown fathers, two were paternal orphans with unknown mothers and three of them were double orphans.

The population of orphaned children in Tembisa is very high with Tembisa Child and Family Welfare Society recording a number of more than 3000 families every year. The average dependency ratio in most of these families is 1:3. In all cases reported to the organization, of every 10 children, eight are orphans affected or infected by HIV and AIDS. Furthermore, amongst 13 participants who were in the focus group discussions, there were three child-care workers and 10 caregivers. All of the participants were female black Africans. The participants' ages ranged from the age of 21–65 years. Two social workers were also interviewed as key informants.

5.2. Challenges faced by HIV and AIDS orphans

The study aimed at investigating the challenges that were being faced in the provision of psychosocial support to HIV and AIDS orphans and the results of these are highlighted in this section.

5.2.1. Theme one: poor health

HIV and AIDS has in the past presented a continuum of complex health issues that ranged from protecting personal health to ensuring that societies have adequate supplies of health care. In Tembisa, the main hospital (Tembisa Hospital) has a facility specifically for children infected with HIV and AIDS. All the children participating in the study who were on anti-retro viral medication or immune boosters claimed to attend *check-ups* at the hospital (Masakhane clinic). Child F stated:

> I started taking Anti Retro Viral treatment at the age of 5 (now 15 years old). It has been a routine for me and they are now like a part of me. My aunt usually takes me to the clinic for my check-up, but when she is not available to do so I go on my own…

Caregivers reported to understand the need to keep the children under constant monitoring to ensure that they did not default on their medication. It was, however, an agreement with most of the participants in the focus group that keeping track of what the children ate and did during school hours was difficult. They reported that because these are children and they like to experiment, they eat most of the things that they are told not to eat at the hospital. They eat these things behind the caregivers' backs. Such defaults only come to light when the children's viral loads spiral after hospital check-up.

Furthermore, the caregivers mentioned that they could not afford nutritious food to give the children. The two social workers who were interviewed also highlighted that the health of orphans deteriorated at times because of lack of nutritious food to eat which is required by those who were living with the virus. One of the social workers said:

> When we send the children for assessments to our doctor or the nurses here, we usually find out that the child's health would have deteriorated in terms of their CD4 count. This is usually caused by the children not eating the right food they are supposed to eat for example vegetables and fruits. (Social Worker 1)

5.2.2. Theme two: inadequate shelter

Of all the children in the study, five reported to be residing in either '*shacks*' or as tenants in outside rooms. Four children reported to be staying in their parental homes and three reported that they lived in the homes of extended family members and that their parents never owned houses of their own. One child stated that:

> I live with my three siblings in my grandmother's house. My mother used to live with us before she fell sick and passed away. Lucky for us, we are the only family my grandmother has now. (Child D)

For most of these children, though the case is quite different and another child highlighted that:

> My aunt has four children of her own and they are girls. She and my mother stayed together in our shack from the time I was born. The shack is two roomed and had one bedroom which my aunt and cousins sleep in. Two of my cousins now have children… there is hardly any space… (Child H).

5.2.3. Theme three: poor school performance

The loss of a parent due to any disease is not easy for a child. Losing a parent to HIV and AIDS is not easy for most children as they suffer from psychosocial effects and often lose concentration at school. Seven of the children interviewed were aware that their parents died of HIV and AIDS and two of these witnessed the illness and death of their parents. Child B reported:

> I was twelve and the eldest. I would help to wash and dress my mother. She was very sick but did not want to go to the hospital until it was too late… She passed away at home in my presence (sobs)…

The child reported that during the time her mother was sick, she went to school occasionally so as to help look after her. Her performance at school dropped a lot that she had to repeat some grades. Four years later, she still remembered the death of her mother like it was yesterday.

In all the interviews, the children indicated that when their parents had the HIV- and AIDS-related sicknesses, their performances in school were affected. Four of the participants suffered through absenteeism from school and hence missed out on some lessons and important tests. Others (six) had to drop out of school after the death of their parents and re-start at a later stage in a new school with present caregivers. Some (two) because of family circumstances were forced to enter into the system and be institutionalized, hence resulting in stigmatization by other learners in those schools. These and other factors have resulted in lower performance by most HIV and AIDS orphans as well as the overburden placed on caregivers to address their needs.

The caregivers also highlighted that the children's performance at school were poor. One caregiver mentioned that:

> At one point I was called by the principal of the school because of the poor performance of my sister's child I am staying with. The principal mentioned that the child was so brilliant but after the death of her mother her grades were getting lower and lower (Caregiver AA)

5.2.4. Theme four: food insecurity

Health and nutrition statuses tend to decline as less money is often available to properly feed the household. One caregiver reported that the greatest challenge they had with caring

http://dx.doi.org/10.5772/66652

for the orphans was that it was not easy having an extra mouth to feed with the present day economy. She stated that:

> I have five children of my own and when my brother died, his three children came to stay with me as his wife died too and I am the only family left. Two of his children are attending school and the youngest is at crèche... my salary was not enough to feed and clothe my children (Caregiver BB)

Through the organization's Family Preservation programme, many community children find a source of food security from the food parcels handed out every month. Normally, family preservation is meant to work with a family for at least 6 months and discharge afterwards. One social worker stated this:

> Some of our clients are placed on family preservation as a temporary measure whilst we work on processing their foster care applications which normally take longer than a year (Social Worker 2).

Tembisa is not an agrarian region; hence farming for food is not an option for many caregivers. None of the community members in the focus groups reported to have a backyard garden in their homes as they claimed that space was taken up by outside rooms which they used as a source of income.

Child B reported that she and her siblings stayed with their parents in the rural areas of Limpopo where life was simple and much cheaper. After the death of their mother, they had to move to Tembisa to stay with their maternal aunt as she was the only surviving family they knew. She described life in Gauteng (Tembisa to be precise) as very expensive as their aunt had to put food on the table every day, clothe them, pay bills and school fees. When asked how they survived, one care giver said that, 'We wait a long time to have foster care grants paid out and most of us are unemployed and survive on part time jobs that give us less than R500.00 a month...'

Another caregiver also highlighted that, '... if it were not for the outside rooms I built from a loan I got from the bank last year, life would be very hard for us... Rental money from tenants helps us...'. For most orphans, the loss of parents meant no more income in the house.

6. Discussion

The aim of the paper was to explore the challenges faced by HIV and AIDS orphans in Tembisa. The data obtained in the study is aligned with the literature which portrays orphan-related challenges which are impacting on the daily lives of the HIV/AIDS-affected and -infected orphans. Notably, the participants' narratives suggested that there were challenges in terms of health, shelter, education and food. According to [27], the death of a parent signifies the disruption of the basic pattern of a child's life. With death comes the challenge of meeting the child's basic needs.

The study highlights that the HIV/AIDS pandemic leaves a trajectory of orphans under the care of overloaded elderly women to assume an inexplicably major role in societal provisions, while undermining their engagement in civil society. This relates to what was outlined that many orphans are being cared for by the already structurally marginalized women, particularly elderly grandmothers often living in destitution [1].

The extended family network that has traditionally existed in Africa and South Africa is finding itself increasingly under strain because of HIV/AIDS [28]. The Department of Social Development in 2012 outlined that the HIV and AIDS pandemic has disrupted family, community and social structures, and has led to a marked increase in the number of orphans and other vulnerable children. The findings of the study strongly support the available literature that argues that children orphaned by HIV and AIDS depend mainly on their extended families to meet their basic needs.

In the case of infected children, their health is determined by the nutrition they get and getting access to their treatments at the right times. Lack of proper finances was found to be a big challenge as most caregivers were either unemployed or at the age of pension. The findings further suggest that although the government has placed certain supports such as social assistance grants, their inaccessibility makes it hard for caregivers to support HIV and AIDS orphans. Increasing poverty can cause a degradation of the immediate family environment and increases health risks whilst reducing its ability to obtain health services [29].

The results of the study also showed that the education of the orphans is disrupted. As [30] put it across, the loss of a productive family member is likely to be a financial burden and might push a family into poverty, increasing the likelihood that a child orphaned by AIDS will miss out on school. More literature confirms this, that, educationally, as poverty and HIV/AIDS reinforce each other, many orphans are denied the right to an education [31, 32]. UNICEF [33] showed that children orphaned by AIDS may miss out on school enrolment, have their schooling interrupted or perform poorly in school as a result of their situation. However, the figures released in 2013 by UNICEF revealed that in most countries in sub-Saharan Africa, the gap between school attendance of orphans and non-orphans has significantly narrowed, although progress varies across the region.

The study indicates that the physiological needs of the orphans are not being met. As Maslow's hierarchy of needs outline, if the physiological needs are not met, the human body cannot function properly and will ultimately fail. These needs are thought to be the most important; they should be met first. Therefore, the plight of orphans could be addressed in the same manner where their basic needs are met for them to get fulfilled.

Since the year 2002, there have been a diverse set of problems associated with the use of the foster care system to provide financial assistance to the country's increasing number of orphans [34]. There has been evidence that the social worker and court-based foster care system are not coping with the demand for foster care orders. In May 2011, the North Gauteng High Court ordered the Department of Social Development to design a comprehensive legal solution to the foster care crisis by 2014 [35]. This was due to the fact that a large number of Foster Care Grants had lapsed by 2009 leaving vulnerable children without assistance while social workers were unable to provide quality services to abused children due to higher foster care caseloads. At the same time, caregivers and children had to wait an unreasonably long time for their grants to be processed. Nevertheless, there has been criticism on the Department of Social Development for a slow and limited response to the crisis in the foster care system [36].

The current Foster Care Grant system demands that the applicant produces both parent's death certificates and affidavit stating who they are in relation to the child and why they are applying for the grant. It is with no reasonable doubt that some orphans are left in the care of extended relatives and grandmothers who have no clue who the fathers or sometimes mothers of the children are. Most of the orphaned children are left without birth registrations and caregivers face problems when trying to register the births of the children. While the access to the Child Support Grants has increased substantially over the years, the Foster Care Grant remains a favourable option for those who can access it because it is more than three times the amount of Child Support Grants [37].

Research by the Children's Institute demonstrates that the extension of the Child Support Grants to all children can play a critical role in supporting children through the AIDS pandemic in South Africa [38]. It argued that the current financial assistance offered by government to orphans (namely the Foster Care Grant) is inappropriate and inadequate in the face of HIV and AIDS because the number of foster care cases in many parts of South Africa already exceeds the capacity of social workers and courts. As a result, many orphans are unable to access Foster Care Grants. This is the case as Tembisa Child and Family Welfare Society where families have to wait a year or two before their applications are processed. At the time of processing, some children are already deceased or the prospective foster parents themselves. In other cases, the children end up moving to other areas as the prospective foster parents cannot afford to provide for them.

Even after the government has allowed for extension orders for foster care to be extended until the child turns 18 and not every 2 years, there is still many social workers and courts are facing in the bid to make foster care applications much faster for clients [39]. The continued use of the administratively complex foster care system for the provision of basic financial support for orphans brings the child protection system to its knees rendering it even less able to provide protection to children who really need it.

The Children's Institute further noted that the poverty of children is neither synonymous with nor exclusive to orphanhood [34]. According to them, a social security system, which provides grants to orphans under the age of 18 without providing adequate support to many other impoverished children whose parents are alive, is simply discriminatory. In other words, it fails to make provisions for the multitude of other children growing up in vulnerability due to HIV and AIDS. There are many South African children growing in the care of HIV- and AIDS-infected mothers or fathers and receive no social support from the state [40]. Their vulnerability is therefore not taken into consideration because one of the parents is still alive.

7. Conclusions and recommendations

Almost three decades into the HIV/AIDS pandemic, most people have an understanding of how AIDS-related deaths impact families [41]. From the discussion of the findings, it can be safely concluded that HIV and AIDS orphans in Tembisa face many challenges in terms of health, education, food and shelter. This means that the physiological needs of these orphans are not met. The fight for the impact of HIV and AIDS is far from being won even though the world has three decades of living in the era of this pandemic. There is therefore a need to provide for ongoing support systems for HIV and AIDS orphans.

While the broader literature confirms that extended families play an important role in care, other data highlight a high level of strain felt by carers. The findings show that caregivers themselves are struggling with dealing with the HIV and AIDS pandemic as they themselves are carriers who also have to deal with the loss of their children or parents, and are left with the burden of caring for orphans. The burden becomes unbearable because most of the caregivers are unemployed and those that are employed make a low income and have other dependents to care for. Accessing state assistance is sometimes a major problem as some orphans are left without birth registrations. Those that do get the assistance are either finding it not enough or as argued by researchers are misusing it. Therefore, the following recommendations are suggested:

- There is an urgent need for kinship caregivers to be given greater support, both financially and emotionally.
- Keeping the orphans and vulnerable children in education should remain a key role of the child care advocates.
- Health education to improve the orphans' knowledge of the dangers they put themselves in when they do not leave a healthy lifestyle. If HIV- and AIDS-infected children are taught how to live healthy lifestyles the re-occurrence of orphanhood due to HIV and AIDS could be stopped. Furthermore, a healthy lifestyle means a long, fruitful life, hence caregivers do not have to go through the pain of losing the children like they did the parents of the children.
- There should be interventions designed to address structural factors such as administration of the Foster Care Grant which may improve outcomes for both caregivers and children.
- Finally, interventions directed at families should take into account the abilities, needs and challenges faced by different types of caregiver, rather than generalizing such that food and shelter needs can be met.

8. Limitations of the study

Due to the purpose of the research, participants might have overemphasized their situation in a hope that the researcher might bring quality services in due course. On the other hand, the participants might have given socially acceptable answers in order to hide their situation and thereby distorting the data that were being collected. Also the fact that one of the researchers was part of the Tembisa Child and Family Welfare Society's social workers might have influenced some responses to be biased. However, the researchers had an informed consent with the participants whereby the aim and objectives of the study were clearly laid

http://dx.doi.org/10.5772/66652

out. The participants were informed that the research was for academic purposes, hence the biasness was limited. This also developed trustworthiness among the participants as they were assured of privacy and confidentiality. The time frame of the research was also a limitation. Regarding the small sample that was used for the study, the findings are not conclusive and cannot be used to make generalizations about the population of interest. However, they develop an initial understanding and sound base for further decision-making.

Author details

Pius Tangwe Tanga*, Princess Khumalo and Priscilla Gutura

*Address all correspondence to: ptanga@ufh.ac.za

University of Fort Hare, Alice, South Africa

References

[1] Joint United Nations Programme on HIV/AIDS. The Gap Report. In. Geneva, Switzerland: UNAIDS; 2014.

[2] Statistics South Africa. Mid-year population estimates. [Internet]. 2015. Available from: http://beta2.statssa.gov.za/publications/P0302/P03022015.pdf [Accessed 2016-02-15].

[3] UNAIDS. Report on the global HIV/AIDS epidemic. [Internet] 2000. Available from http://data.unaids.org/pub/Report/2000/2000_gr_en.pdf [Accessed 2015-10-30].

[4] UNICEF. Measuring the Determinants of Childhood Vulnerability [internet]. 2014. Available from: http://data.unicef.org/hiv-aids/care-support [Accessed 2015-11-23].

[5] Nyangara F, Kalungwa Z, Obiero W, Thurman TR, Chapman J. Promoting a home-based program model for supporting children affected by HIV/AIDS: Evaluation of Tumaini project in Iringa region, Tanzania. MEASURE Evaluation. 2009.

[6] Kawewe SM. Reclaiming civil society and the plight of AIDS orphaned children and elderly women caregivers in sub-Saharan Africa: a global human rights dilemma for international social workers. Women in Welfare Education. 2006 Nov 1; 8:64–77.

[7] September R, Dinbabo M. Gearing up for implementation: A new Children's Act for South Africa. Practice. 2008; 1: 20(2):113–122.

[8] White Paper. Principles, guidelines, recommendations, proposed policies and programmes for developmental social welfare in South Africa. Republic of South Africa: Department of Welfare. 1997.

[9] South African Social Security Agency (SASSA). Statistical report on social grants. [Internet] 2016. Available from: www.sassa.gov.za [Accessed 2016-05-02].

[10] Leibbrandt M, Woolard I, Finn A, Argent J. Trends in South African income distribution and poverty since the fall of apartheid. 2010.

[11] Pauw K, Mncube L. Expanding the social security net in South Africa: Opportunities, challenge and constraints. Development Policy Research Unit (DPRU). Working Paper 07/127. University of Cape Town; 2007.

[12] Sowetan. Misuse of social grants is rife. [Internet] 2012. Available from: http://www.sowetanlive.co.za/news/2012/05/25/misuse-of-social-grants-is-rife [Accessed 2015-10-28].

[13] Barnes H, Noble M, Wright G, Dawes A. A geographical profile of child deprivation in South Africa. Child Indicators Research. 2009; 2:181–199. DOI: 10.1007/s12187-008-9026-2

[14] Wright G, Barnes H, Noble M, Dawes A. The South African index of multiple deprivation for children 2001 at database level. Pretoria: Department of Social Development. 2009.

[15] Kirby D, Laris BA, Rolleri L. Sex and HIV education programs for youth: their impact and important characteristics. 2006.

[16] Joint United Nations Programme on HIV/AIDS. Report on the Global Acquired Immunodeficiency Syndrome Epidemic. UNAIDS; 2008.

[17] Children's Institute. Analysis of the 2009/10 budgets of the nine provincial departments of Social Development: Are the budgets adequate to implement the Children's Act? [Internet]. 2009. Available from http://www.ci.org.za/depts/ci/pubs/pdf/rights/workpap/Childrens_Act_Budget_Analyss_2009_Prov_DSD_Votes_28May2009.pdf [Accessed 2015-08-25].

[18] Meintjies H, Hall K. Child Rights in Focus. University of Cape Town Children's Institute, CapeTown. 2009.

[19] Bradshaw D, Johnson L, Schneider H, Bourne D, Dorrington R. Orphans of the HIV/AIDS Epidemic. Burden of Disease Research Unit, Medical Research Council. 2002:1–4.

[20] Twine R, Collinson M A, Polzer-Ngwato T, Kahn K. Evaluating access to a child-oriented poverty alleviation intervention in Rural South Africa. Scandinavian Journal of Public Health. 2007; 35:118–127. DOI: 10.1080/14034950701430008

[21] Kaseke E. The role of social security in South Africa. Social Work. 2010; **53**: 159–168. DOI: 10.1177/0020872809355394

[22] Maslow A H. Motivation and Personality. (3rd ed.). New York, NY: Harper & Row. 1987.

[23] Huitt, W. Maslow's hierarchy of needs. Educational Psychology Interactive. Valdosta, GA: Valdosta State University. [Internet] 2007. Available from http://www.edpsycinteractive.org/topics/regsys/maslow.html [Accessed 2015-08-25].

[24] The Adler Group. Maslow's hierarchy of hiring pyramid: performance based hiring. [Internet] 2011. Available from: http://www.eremedia.com/ere/maslows-hierarchy-of-hiring-pyramid-according-to-adler/[Accessed 2015-10-31].

[25] Creswell JW. An Introduction to Qualitative Research. London: Sage; 2008.

[26] De Vos AS, Strydom H, Fouche CB, Delcourt SSL. Research at Grass Roots for the Social Science and Human Service Professions. 3rd edition. Pretoria: Van Schaick Publishers; 2005.

[27] Gambril E. Research on Social Work Practice. Englewood Cliffs, NJ: Prentice Hall; 2010.

[28] Ferreira M. HIV/AIDS and family well-being in Southern Africa: Towards an analysis of policies and responsiveness. United Nations Department of Economic and Social Affairs Division for Social Policy and Development Policy. Windhoek, Namibia. 2015.

[29] Nyawasha TS. Psychosocial Support to Orphans and Vulnerable Children. Word-mart. [Internet] 2006. Available from http://www.wordmart.com/html/psycho-social_support1.html [Accessed 2015-09-05].

[30] UNICEF, UNAIDS W. UNFPA and UNESCO. Children and AIDS: Fifth Stocktaking Report, 2010, Geneva, Switzerland. 2010.

[31] Lachman P, Poblete X, Ebigbo PO, Nyandiya-Bundy S, Bundy R P, Killian B, Doek J. Challenges facing child protection. Child Abuse and Neglect. 2002; 26:587–617. ISSN: 01452134.

[32] Subbarao K, Coury D. Reaching out to Africa's Orphans: A Framework for Public Action. World Bank Publications; Washington D.C, USA. 2004.

[33] UNICEF. Africa's Orphaned and Vulnerable Generations: Children Affected by AIDS. UNICEF; 2006.

[34] Children's Institute. *South African Child Gauge* [internet]. 2012. Available from: http://www.ci.org.za/depts/ci/pubs/pdf/general/gauge2012/sa_child_gauge2012.pdf (Accessed 2015-10-28).

[35] Proudlock P, Hall K, Meintjies H, Jamieson L. Children's Institute amicus curiae affidavit in Sithasolwazi Stemele & Minister for Social Development, Case No. 14/1/4-206/10, South Gauteng High Court, 2011. Retrieved from: www.ci.org.za.

[36] Business Day Live. NGOs criticise ministerial committee probing Foster Care Grants. [Internet]. 2014. Available from: http://www.bdlive.co.za/national/2014/10/24/ngos-criticise-ministerial-committee-probing-foster-care-grants [Accessed 2015-05-08].

[37] Jacobs M, Shung-King M, Smith C, editors. South African child gauge 2005. Children's Institute, University of Cape Town; 2005.

[38] Avert Organization. HIV and AIDS Information [internet]. 2004. Available from: www.avert.org. [Accessed 2015-11-20].

[39] Gray M. Back to basics: A critique of the strengths perspective in social work. Families in Society: The Journal of Contemporary Social Services. 2011 Jan 1; 92(1):5–11.

[40] Rosa S, Guthrie T. Extending the child support grant to all children under 18 years. ACCESS, Children's Institute, UCT. 2002.

[41] Kuo C, Operario D. Caring for AIDS orphaned children: An exploratory study of the challenges faced by carers in KZN, South Africa. Vulnerable Child Youth Studies. 2010; 5:344–352. DOI: 10.1080/17450128.2010.516372

Chapter 5

Difficulties and Coping Strategies Experienced by Employed People with HIV in Japan: A Qualitative Study Comparing High and Low Sense of Coherence Groups

Tomoko Omiya, Yoshihiko Yamazaki,
Megumi Shimada, Kazuko Ikeda,
Seiko Ishiuchi-Ishitani and Katsumi Ohira

Additional information is available at the end of the chapter

http://dx.doi.org/10.5772/65775

Abstract

People with HIV experience anxiety about discrimination in the workplace and disclosing their disease. Effective coping ability toward HIV-related challenges may be associated with a person's sense of coherence (SOC). This study describes the range of difficulties HIV-positive individuals experience and their coping strategies, especially in the workplace. The experiences of those with high and low SOC are compared. Data were collected in Japan from 2007 to 2009 using a qualitative approach. Semistructured interviews were conducted with 40 participants with HIV with work experience. Interviews focused on individual's perspectives, including self-perceptions of physical and mental functioning, work conditions, and perceived changes in their circumstances. Participants were divided into high and low SOC groups based on SOC-13 scores. A number of categories and subcategories of experiences were extracted, including "acute feeling of the severe social positioning of HIV," with some categories specific to those with low SOC. Those with high SOC appeared to have a unique perspective that supported more successful coping, for example, "Awareness of death is linked to valuing living in the present," "Do not be discouraged by uncertainties and difficulties," and so on. It suggests that development of coping skills may help people with HIV.

Keywords: coping strategies, qualitative study, salutogenesis, sense of coherence, Japan

1. Introduction

Acquired immunodeficiency syndrome (AIDS) is characterized by infection with human immunodeficiency virus (HIV) and serious, systemic dysfunction of immunity. Although its global incidence rate is declining, the rate of HIV infection is increasing in Japan, reaching approximately 16,000 cases in 2014 [1]. In the last decade, new treatments for HIV infection and AIDS have improved health and life expectancy for many people who are HIV-positive. In the recent era of highly active antiretroviral therapy, the estimated median survival for a young person diagnosed with HIV infection is >35 years [2]. Most people with HIV are in a stable and manageable condition [3], with this group accounting for the majority of people infected with HIV in Japan, particularly males aged 20–40 years. For this group, infection was diagnosed at a time critical for career development [1].

The importance of employment has been emphasized in many studies on chronic diseases [4]. Employment helps people to function as adults and find self-worth, therefore playing an important role in maintaining human dignity [5]. Mental health is reported to be better in people with HIV who are employed than in those who are unemployed [6]. However, in the workplace, people with HIV suffer from anxiety about discrimination and layoff [7]. Disclosing the name of their disease may also be highly problematic for them [8, 9].

In many life situations, people with HIV experience various stressors [10]; for example, HIV is perceived as a more stigmatized disease than cancer [11]. People with HIV are also faced with problems unique to HIV, which further affect their vulnerability and makes psychological adjustment more difficult [12]. People with HIV are, therefore, forced to cope with highly stressful situations, brought about by stigma and their own anxiety about experiencing stigma.

Sense of coherence (SOC), a concept proposed by the health sociologist Antonovsky, was conceptualized and standardized as the ability to cope successfully [13]. SOC focuses on salutary factors (i.e., health factors) described as "salutogenesis" [14]. Rather than focusing on pathogenesis, or a conventional medical line of questioning regarding the causes of disease, salutogenesis aims to shed light on what creates health.

Antonovsky created the salutogenic model, which illustrates relationships among stressors, coping (tension coping and coping resources), and SOC. The salutogenic model comprises two theoretical models. First, in the face of stressors and the resulting strain, SOC copes by mobilizing generalized resistance resources. The success or failure of coping depends on the richness of coping resources and the strength of SOC. The second theoretical model explains that SOC is formed by good life experiences and strengthened by successful experiences of coping with tension. The quality of these good life experiences is formed by "generalized resistance resources" (GRRs) [13]. GRRs can be identified as resources bound to an individual's capacities and include material and nonmaterial qualities ranging from individual level factors to those of the person's culture and/or society [15]. That is, GRRs are the physical, biological, artifactual-material, cognitive, emotional, valuative-attitudinal, interpersonal-relational, and macro-sociocultural characteristics of an individual or a group that are effective in avoiding or combating a wide variety of stressors [14].

The salutogenic model indicates that success or failure of stress coping depends on the level of SOC. Higher SOC brings more successful coping, which results in further strengthening SOC. Therefore, a positive spiral relationship has been suggested between SOC and successful coping experiences. In other words, high SOC helps stress coping, which promotes redefinition and reconstruction of the experience, creating a virtuous cycle [14, 15].

Describing coping experiences of people with high SOC is to describe successful coping with stressors. It is also important to describe how flexibly and successfully those with high SOC are able to cope. This may lead to useful suggestions for supporting people with HIV. In addition, comparing different coping styles of people with HIV who have high or low SOC, and examining their unique experiences and living environments may provide clues to their different perspectives and coping behaviors. Particular difficulties experienced by a person with HIV may also be related to low SOC or a decline in SOC.

There is a lack of information on the appropriate types of workplace support for people with HIV in the workforce. The present study aimed to describe the difficulties and coping strategies experienced by people with HIV in the workplace and compare the experiences of those with high and low SOC using the 13-item SOC scale [16]. It is anticipated that the results may provide clues to appropriate types of workplace support for people with HIV.

2. Method

2.1. Study design

Antonovsky stated that qualitative studies are useful to better understand the function of SOC, including its strength and flexibility [13]. The present study wanted to examine participants' experiences from their perspectives and analyze their work life from a new standpoint based on the salutogenic model. A qualitative approach was considered appropriate for these goals.

2.2. Participant recruitment

First, medical facilities with specialized HIV outpatient clinics in Tokyo were asked to invite patients to participate in the study; 15 patients were recruited in total. Inclusion criteria were patients in their twenties to early fifties whose symptoms had been stabilized and who had work experience. Participants were recruited by nurses when visiting the facilities for treatment. Participants chose where the interviews took place, with most taking place at the medical facilities. NPO corporations and social welfare corporations were also contacted and asked to assist with recruitment of participants, and a further 25 participants were recruited. This second round of recruitment increased the diversity of the sampling routes as access to participants living in different areas (Kansai and Kyushu) was made possible. Three pilot interviews and the first 15 interviews for the present study were conducted by two interviewers. The interviewers were the first author and a researcher with a medical degree (Seiko Ishiuchi-Ishitani, fifth author) who was familiar with the interview questions and had worked as a special consultant for a social welfare corporation offering assistance to people with HIV. These interviews were conducted by two interviewers because the purpose of the present study was to collect explorative data, and it was considered beneficial to observe participants from multiple angles. It was also thought that the presence of an interviewer who was affiliated with a social welfare corporation assisting people with HIV may give participants a sense of security and facilitate development of rapport. The 25 interviews in the latter half of the study were conducted by the first author only. The question items were more narrowly focused and based on the earlier data, and as participants introduced by the medical facilities were cooperative, no problems arising from one interviewer were anticipated. During the analysis of participant interviews, it became clear that the results would need to be further evaluated depending on infection route (homosexual contact, heterosexual contact, and tainted blood products), sex, type of employment (regular or irregular), and progression to AIDS. Therefore, it was decided that throughout the study, interviews would cover people with diverse characteristics. As the majority of patients infected through homosexual contact were men, female patients and patients infected by tainted blood products were considered to have different experiences. Therefore, these patients were invited to participate at slightly higher rates than the actual infection rate. We stopped recruiting participants after the number of interviews reached 40, as this was deemed to have reached saturation. Participant details are shown in **Table 1**.

2.3. Data collection

During recruitment and on the day of the interview, participants were assured of privacy through verbal explanations and in written documentation. Before their interview began, participants signed a consent form that included permission to record the interview. The interviews took place in situations where privacy was secured, such as conference rooms and training rooms at a library. The interview duration ranged from 40 to 135 min, with a mean duration of 75 min. Interviews were conducted from September 2007 to September 2009. The interview questions covered: participants' perspectives of their physical and mental functioning since HIV infection was identified, working conditions and the type of job at the time, reactions of people around them, disclosure of infection, relationship with a partner, what HIV means to them, whether their views about HIV and feelings about life and work had changed, what kinds of change occurred, and how they evaluated these changes. The interview was particularly focused on participants' ways of thinking, asking "Why did you behave that way? (or not behave that way)"; "What does the experience mean to you?"; and "Why did you think that way?"

2.4. SOC scale

We used the 13-item, 5-point version of the SOC scale, because the interviews were expected to take a long time and to allow comparison with survey data from a nationwide representative sample [16]. The reliability validity of SOC-13 Japanese edition was determined in a randomly selected nationwide sample of 1800 men and women aged over 20 years. The SOC mean for the sample was 44.06 ± 8.83 [16].

2.5. Ethical considerations

The first author has significant experience working as an occupational health nurse, as well as in supporting people who have a disease that is difficult to disclose to others; this breadth

http://dx.doi.org/10.5772/65775

	n	%
Demographics		
Gender		
Male	35	87.5
Female	5	12.5
Age group		
<30	5	12.5
30 ≤ 39	17	42.5
40 ≤ 49	15	37.5
50 ≤ 59	3	7.5
Education		
University, graduate school	18	45.0
Junior/high school and other	13	32.5
No answer	9	22.5
HIV-associated indicators		
The length of time since HIV diagnose		
<1 year	0	0.0
1–4 years	15	37.5
5–10 years	12	30.0
11 years and above	13	32.5
Route of HIV infection		
Tainted blood products and blood transfusion	5	12.5
Sexual contact	34	85.0
Unknown	1	2.5
CD4 cell counts		
200 ≤ 500/μl	19	47.5
500/μl≤	21	52.5
Sexuality		
Heterosexual	10	25.0
Homosexual	24	60.0
Bisexual	6	15.0

Table 1. Demographic characteristics of participants ($n = 40$).

of experience enhanced understanding of the difficulties in interpersonal relationships in the workplace. After consulting with the facilities several times, careful consideration was given to the protection of privacy, participants' physical condition at the time of the interview, and arrangement of a comfortable interview place for participants. The purpose of the study, methods, protection of privacy, and disclosure of the results were explained to participants orally and in writing. Participants were informed that they would be able to participate with a fictitious name, to ask any questions during the interview, would not have to answer if they did not want to, and would be able to stop participating at any point. Participants recruited through medical facilities were informed that the interviewer was not associated with the facilities and that their treatment would not be affected in any way, even if they withdrew from participation. The recordings, verbatim transcripts, and analysis notes were stored in a locked room, and the data were stored with real names and other personal information converted into codes. These materials could only be accessed with a password.

The present study was approved by the Medical Research Ethics Committee of Tokyo University, Graduate School (Approval No. 2403), and the Ethics Committee of the National Center for Global Health and Medicine (Approval No. 675).

2.6. Analysis

2.6.1. Interview data

The method of Lofland [17] was used to analyze interview data. First, a transcript of the interview was read repeatedly to grasp the whole picture of the interview. The information was then coded, categorized, and analyzed, with reference to the results of intergroup comparisons between participants with high and low SOC. To ensure the validity of the results, discussions and member checking were conducted with coresearchers [18].

2.6.2. Measuring SOC

SOC was measured after the interview. With the permission of participants, responses were collected while the interview was still being recording, and the majority of their responses were confirmed. According to Söderhamn is collect! [19], an official cut-off point is not prescribed for SOC, and the cut-off point differed in quantitative studies comparing high and low SOC [20, 21]. In qualitative research, the SOC score analysis cannot be conducted by performing group division. However, there is an exception in a study conducted in Croatia [22] that used the SOC-29 (7-point scale), which is the most commonly used version globally. In our study, we used the SOC-13 (5-point scale), as we intended to divide participants based on Japanese mean score. No previous research is available about group division of the SOC-13. Therefore, this was discussed among the present researchers while referring to a Japanese average score. Participants' average SOC-13 score was 43.0 ± 7.9. Given that the scale ranged from 13 to 60, this score was slightly higher than the nationwide sample average (the average score was 41.15 for those in their thirties and 42.16 for those in their forties) [16]. Based on the average score, median score, scores from previous studies, and the nationwide sample scores, participants scoring over 42 (n = 22) were categorized as the high SOC group, with those scoring 39 or less (n = 12) defined as the low SOC group. The remaining six participants scored 40–42 and were categorized as the middle SOC group.

http://dx.doi.org/10.5772/65775

3. Results

3.1. Difficulties faced by participants

In the present paper, [ ] indicates a category, << >> a sub-category, and < > a code. Relevant quotations from the interviews have been included to illustrate key themes. Details in parentheses after the quotations indicate the participant's ID number, sex, and SOC score (range 13–65).

Difficulties experienced by participants were divided into three domains: physical, social, and personal. Physical domain categories were [Awareness of death] and [Low possibility of maintaining one's physical condition]. Social (employment, interpersonal) domain categories were [Inability to maintain or weakening of coherence with respect to work], [Being made aware of the lack of understanding and knowledge about HIV in society], [Cut off from society because of the name of the illness], and [Keeping love and marriage at a distance]. The personal domain was represented by the categories [Feelings of guilt and self-reproach] and [Having complicated feelings about being infected]. No distinctive difficulties were observed in the high SOC group.

3.1.1. Difficulties specific to patients with low SOC

Four distinctive subcategories found in the low SOC group were the following: <<Being at work becomes difficult after infection is determined>>; <<Leaving one's job due to the fear of HIV becoming known>>; <<Being seized by the idea that working hard has no meaning>>; and <<Just getting by is enough for my life>> (**Table 2**).

> *I don't find any meaning in working so hard. To be honest, I just think it's enough to do whatever is in front of me. That's the only prospect I have at the moment. (#31, male, score: 33)*

Some participants in the low SOC group experienced [Being made to realize the lack of understanding and knowledge about HIV in society].

> *During a job interview, people ask how I got the disease. My answer is "because I had sex without using a condom." They probably don't understand much about immunodeficiency, even people who want to hire people to whom the Disabled People Employment Promotion Act applies.(#9, male, score: 34)*

In the category [Cut off from society because of the name of the illness], participants in the low SOC group reported experiencing severe stigma, including: <<Being told that my handicap isn't normal>> and <<Being told that you don't get that disease if you live a normal life>>. Participants reported that stigma by people they were close to and had a good relationship with in the workplace or where they received treatment was most hurtful. This stigma was particularly felt when a participant was hired under the Disabled People Employment Promotion Act, and for some, this became a major reason to give up working.

> *(As a worker covered by the Disabled People Employment Promotion Act) when I was having my individual counseling, the first thing they said was "we didn't want to hire you from the start." Loud and clear. Looking back now, the president of the company must have told them to hire me. They perhaps couldn't say no and hired me unwillingly. They even told me, "We wanted to employ a normal disabled person, so to speak." (#43, male, score: 28)*

Domain	**Categories**	**Subcategories** **Difficulties peculiar to patients with low SOC**
Physical	[Awareness of death] [Low possibility of maintaining one's physical condition]	
Social (employment, interpersonal)	[Inability to maintain/weakening of coherence with respect to work]	<<Being at work becomes difficult after infection is determined>> <<Leaving one's job due to the fear of HIV becoming known>> <<Being seized by the idea that working hard is no meaning>> <<Just getting by is enough for my life>>
	[Being made to realize the lack of understanding and knowledge about HIV in society] low SOC only	<<Being asked that why you were infected>> <<Being asked the meaning of immune dysfunction>>
	[Cut off from society by virtue of the disease's name]	<< Being told that my handicap isn't normal>> <<Being told that you don't get that disease if you live a normal life>>
	[Keeping love and marriage at a distance]	<<Arguments about who gave who the infection with partner>>
		<<A poor relationship with a lover or a partner>>
Personal	[Feelings of guilt and self-reproach] [Having complicated feelings about being infected]	<<Victims who had been infected by someone else>> <<Anger towards the person who passed on the infection>>

Table 2. Difficulties experienced by participants

Besides difficulties at work, participants experienced anguish on an interpersonal level about disclosure of their infection to significant others and about lovers and marriage. Particularly in the low SOC group, participants felt there were <<Arguments about who gave who the infection>> which led to <<A poor relationship with a lover or a partner>>, and as a result they (sexually infected homosexual males) experienced [Keeping love and marriage at a distance].

> *The person I was going out with had shingles twice in a row. Then I thought I could also have it (HIV) and so I checked. He probably gave it to me, but he didn't tell me anything. In the end, I lost my trust in him and we broke up. (#31, male, score: 33)*

Participants expressed [Feelings of guilt and self-reproach] for having become infected; particularly, participants in the low SOC group felt very strongly that they could not understand and accept why they had been infected. As a result, they perceived themselves as <<Victims who had been infected by someone else>>. This feeling of being a victim was linked to <<Anger towards the person who passed on the infection>> who they felt was to blame.

I trusted the pitcher (the person who inserts his penis) and didn't wear a rubber. That's how I got it, and the guilty party, so to speak, was my partner and he is responsible. I can't forgive him for that. (#43, male, score: 28)

3.2. Characteristic coping experiences in the high SOC group

Coping experiences characteristic of the high SOC group are presented in **Table 3**.

These experiences were classified by encounter environment and way of coping. In terms of the environment, employment and personal relationships were extracted as categories in the social domain. Coping may also be classified as being cognitive or behavioral.

3.2.1. Social domain

In the category [A workplace environment enabling maintenance of coherence with respect to work], working conditions were important, such as access to a paid vacation and a fully equipped welfare system. Other important conditions were no shift work, preservation of privacy, minimal overwork, minimal other physical burdens, and stable work. In addition, <<A workplace climate appreciating diversity>> was important for men who have sex with men. This enabled them to continue doing the same job in the same way as before infection.

In our corporate climate, people don't get involved with each other unless it concerns business. There are quite a few people who take sick leave in my company because of bad physical and mental condition. When they are back in the office, everyone behaves normally as though nothing special has happened. (#39, male, score: 50)

The category [Opportunity to have a workplace where one is needed and where colleagues trust each other] reflected the importance of personal relationships in the workplace. One participant who became infected through sexual contact with another man commented on informing his superior of his need for leave of absence due to the infection.

Since I was infected with HIV, my condition was bad and I decided to tell my superior. When I was about to tell him how I was infected, he said, "Take a rest" and "How you got the disease doesn't matter to me at all. You are still you and I understand very well how hard you have been working." (#4, male, score: 49)

In this way, <<Having the confidence that even though infected, one is still trusted as a member of society>> provided substantial moral support.

The category [Had opportunity to know someone who understands about the infection] indicated understanding of HIV infection by significant others, such as parents and siblings, friends, lovers, and partners. Many participants commented on how, at difficult times, such as the onset of AIDS and when they lost their jobs, they had been helped by others who <<Offered comfort during times of physical and mental stress>>. Among their significant others, it was important that there were <<Friends who remained as close as they had been before hearing of the infection>> and <<Support from the company's occupational health doctor>> in the workplace. However, only participants who were hired because of a disability or who had hemophilia told their company's occupational health doctor about their disease. Even if the company's occupational health doctor said they were thorough about

Domain	Categories	Subcategories	Coping caracteristics
Social (employment, personal relationships)	[A workplace environment enabling maintenance of coherence with respect to work]	<<A workplace climate appreciating diversity>>	Coping whth the environment they encounter
	[Opportunity to have a workplace where one is needed and where colleagues trust each other]	<<Having the confidence that even though infected, one is still trusted as a member of society>>	
	[Had opportunity to know someone who understands about the infection]	<<Offered confort during times of physical and mental stress>> <<Friends who remained as close as they had been before hearing of the infection>> <<Support from the company's occupational health doctor>> <<No change in love and affection from spouse, lover or partner after informing them of the infection>>	
	[The infection provided an opportunity to build/rebuild important bonds]	<<ebuilding relationships with significant others as a result of infection>> <<Infection led to meeting irreplaceable people>>	
	[No perception of direct stigma]	<<The attitude was the same as that towards other disabilities>>	
	[Treat the infection and related events neutrally]	<<Being infected is unlucky but not a disaster>> <<Apart from the infection, I'm happy so it's OK>> <<Everyone faces their own difficulties and anxieties>> <<Is the problem really caused by HIV?>>	Cognitive coping
	[Awareness of death is linked to valuing living in the present]	<<Think about what kind of work I really want to do and how to live>>	
	[Judging and assessing events from a long-term point of view]	<<Particular events in the past resulted in me being in this position now>>	
	[Create boundary lines for important things, do a reality check, and then actively change them]	<<Reaching a compromise between the content and conditions of work and one's physical condition and or environment>> <<Changing one's work goals and aim in life>>	

http://dx.doi.org/10.5772/65775

Domain	Categories	Subcategories	Coping caracteristics
	["Anyway, give it a try" behavior]	<<Disclosed the infection to a partner or lover in an attempt to have them accept it>> <<Disclosure of the infection at the company to gain the support of superiors and colleagues at the workplace>> <<Disclosure of the infection to friends to confirm the way of socializing in the future>> <<Ask for help myself>>	Behavioral coping
	[Do not be discouraged by uncertainties and difficulties]		Cognitive coping
	[Being infected cannot be helped and I am prepared for the worst]	<<I accept responsibility for becoming HIV-infected (infection between homosexuals)>> <<I am not going to be at the mercy of anger due to the infection (harmful effects of medicines, heterosexual)>>	
	[Ready to live one's own life]	<<Live while regretting one's behavior that led to infection (homosexual infection)>> <<I will go straight>>	
		<<Be thoroughly prepared for the onset of AIDS and dying before others>>	

Table 3. Coping experiences observed in high SOC participants

protecting privileged information, many participants did not tell anyone in the company about their HIV infection.

> *The drugs I was taking were no longer suitable for me and I really thought of suicide then. It took me about half a year to get settled, and my mother came regularly from my hometown to stay with me because she thought I shouldn't be left alone. She really helped me a lot.(#23, male, score: 49)*

Almost all participants felt they had to tell their spouse, lover, or partner about their infection to prevent them also becoming infected. In this situation, many participants in the high SOC group experienced <<No change in love and affection from spouse, lover, or partner after informing them of the infection>>. Some received considerable support from the presence of significant others who understood about HIV infection and continued to accept them.

> *I have only dated two people since I found out about my disease. I would tell him/her about my condition (HIV) and ask if he/she is still sure. Interviewer: "And if he/she says it's OK, then the relationship could start?" I would feel that I should do my best for them.(#39, male, score: 50)*

The category [The infection provided an opportunity to build/rebuild important bonds] included the subcategory <<Rebuilding relationships with significant others as a result of infection>>. This was reflected by participants who reported that disclosing HIV infection improved their relationships with other people, particularly parents, siblings, and other blood relatives. Participants in the high SOC group experienced love and affection from their parents and siblings, and felt disclosing the infection provided a chance to rebuild relationships.

> *Since our points of view have been always different, my brother and I weren't so close once we had both grown up. However, because he is younger, my brother was very understanding, and said "anybody could be infected." That changed my relationship with him completely. Now we are very close. If I hadn't been infected, things probably wouldn't have turned out this way. (#26, female, score: 53)*

Another subcategory, <<Infection led to meeting irreplaceable people>>, referred to those who felt lucky because they had met people they would never have met if they had not been infected. As well as attaching a more positive meaning to HIV infection, this was a source of energy for some participants to live with HIV and continue living.

> *Then I met this man and realized that he loved me for everything, including my disease. I thought that even if I never go out with another man until I die, that's OK, because this experience was quite enough for me. Looking back now, I wouldn't have met this man who really loved me if I hadn't had my disease. As he said himself, to find each other I had to have been infected. We wouldn't have shared any common ground, otherwise. (#26, female, score: 53)*

The category [No perception of direct stigma] was common for participants in the high SOC group. These participants reported that regardless of the route of infection, when the name of their disease was disclosed when applying for a job open to disabled people, they experienced <<The attitude was the same as that toward other disabilities>>, and even if there was concern for their physical condition, the attitudes of people around them did not change.

> *The top people of the company weren't prejudiced and the company's philosophy was to let more disabled people have jobs and participate in society. So, I thought I preferred to tell them and be employed. At the interview, they asked me, as they do normally, "Is there any difficulty when you work?" and "Do you visit hospital regularly?" and so on. I told them "There are no problems when I work because my condition is stable." (#10, male, score: 46)*

http://dx.doi.org/10.5772/65775

3.2.2. Cognitive and behavioral coping

3.2.2.1. Cognitive coping

The category [Treat the infection and related events neutrally] reflected how participants in the high SOC group tended to view things objectively and look at them calmly from a distance. This was observed in the high SOC group, where even if participants experienced feeling guilty or depressed, they felt that <<Being infected is unlucky but not a disaster>>. When re-evaluating their current lives, they felt <<Apart from the infection, I'm happy, so it's OK>>. When comparing their past with the present, they thought about past hardships with the infection in the context of <<Everyone faces their own difficulties and anxieties>>.

Some participants also reported that when others knew of the infection, they sometimes reacted negatively. Even without experiencing strong stigma, this response made participants feel bitter, sad, or angry. However, those in the high SOC group reflected on the situation later and wondered <<Is the problem really caused by HIV?>>. They perceived hard experiences as not necessarily all being a result of HIV. They thought objectively about their own HIV infection and looked at themselves with a calm, neutral attitude.

> *Well, it wasn't a friend of mine but an acquaintance of my spouse. She knew about my infection and someone told me that she was talking about me behind my back. Apparently, she said that she didn't want to have meals with me, or something. But of course, that isn't all about my disease. I reckon that's something to do with liking or disliking each other. Me being an HIV carrier is the excuse she uses. She probably just hated my personality (laughs). (#26, female, score: 53)*

The category [Awareness of death is linked to valuing living in the present] reflected how participants assumed there was a high possibility of dying prematurely. Those in the high SOC group were observed to live life to the fullest, do what they wanted to do now, and <<Think about what kind of work I really want to do and how to live>>.

> *It's true that I can work harder since I got this disease. Before, when I was healthy, I had so little motivation. After I got ill, I became very grateful to my company. I became ill and they still employ me. They allow me to take leave, too. Then, I remembered that I really wanted to continue working because when I left my hometown, I made a strong resolution. (#37, male, score: 57)*

The category [Judging and assessing events from a long-term point of view] represented those who considered that <<Particular events in the past resulted in me being in this position now>> rather than making fragmentary judgments or assessments. Furthermore, they reported that "what I am experiencing now will be in some way useful in the future." Inevitably, perceiving that the past, present, and future are joined was linked to comments about belief in invisible powers such as "believing in fate" and "believing in God's will."

> *I got this (HIV) and it had an influence on my field of specialization. I had to give up. I was disappointed, but somehow I was able to think positively that something good would turn up and that this infection must be useful for something in the future. Interviewer: "What made you think so?" I've always been like that. I think positively and believe in what I think (laughs). That's all. (#33, male, score: 44)*

The category [Create boundary lines for important things, do a reality check, and then actively change them] described how, for many participants, HIV infection led to letting go of things that were important or giving up long-term dreams. This was particularly true for work. In the high SOC group, there were some who accepted this, coping by <<Reaching a compromise between the content and conditions of work and one's physical condition and/or environment>> and <<Changing one's work goals and aim in life>>. Being aware that decisions lie within oneself was particularly important. Even if the current situation involved unavoidable reconciliation, awareness that one must make the final decision alone, be confident, and make decisions independently was important.

> *(Because of the infection, this person was transferred to a clerical position from working outside the office) I really wanted to continue the job I was doing until I had gained one year of experience. But, thinking about the trouble I might cause other people if I insisted on doing the former job, and the company's offer of allowing me to continue working, in the end I decided by myself that I should do my best in the new position. (#4, male, employed, score: 49)*

3.2.2.2. Behavioral coping

The category ["Anyway, give it a try" behavior] often applied when infection was disclosed to a lover or a partner. Nearly all participants in the low SOC group had given up the idea of having a lover saying, "After all, I can't make love" and "Nobody would understand." In contrast, participants in the high SOC group reported that they carefully planned the timing and <<Disclosed the infection to a partner or a lover in an attempt to have them accept it>>. This resulted in the relationship continuing in some cases and ending in others. Either way, participants accepted the outcome. In addition to affectionate relationships, there was positive behavior shown by <<Disclosure of the infection at the company to gain the support of superiors and colleagues in the workplace>> and <<Disclosure of the infection to friends to confirm the way of socializing in the future>>. Whether or not infection was disclosed, a "give it a try" attitude was characteristic of the general behavior of many participants, for example, <Ask for help myself>.

> *I learned a lot by asking the doctor at the hospital. "...This medicine works this way so the virus reacts this way and is deactivated." I am given explanations like that so I thoroughly understand. (#39, male, score: 50)*

The category [Do not be discouraged by uncertainties and difficulties] reflected the tendency of participants in the high SOC group to meet challenges even if they had initially failed. One participant disclosed his infection to a person he had become fond of, which ended the relationship. He also disclosed the infection to the next person he came to love, feeling a moral obligation to tell the other party because of the infection risk. Despite the fact that a relationship ending is hurtful, the participant maintained his stance about disclosing infection.

> *Being rejected by the person you want to go out with... I remember three times. Interviewer: "Three times? Did you have any fears about being rejected again (if you disclose the infection)?" Well, it would be a lie if I said no. Interviewer: "After being turned down by several people, don't you feel that you don't want to disclose your infection anymore? Because the person before rejected you, do you think the next person must do the same?" I don't think so. In fact, some people didn't reject me. I don't think that everyone is the same. There are many different people living in this world. (#10, male, score: 56)*

Participants held similar attitudes regarding work. In cases where a participant decided their infection should be disclosed at work, their behavior was to disclose the infection. Even if one company did not hire them, they tried talking to another company about the infection.

3.2.3. High SOC group attitudes as a result of coping

Experiences in the category [Being infected cannot be helped and I am prepared for the worst] differed between the high and low SOC groups. Participants in the low SOC group experienced becoming infected with HIV as "the result of giving in to the demand of the other party (sexual contact without using a condom)" or "due to betrayal by a person I trusted." In contrast, those in the high SOC group felt that "It was my own fault," <<I accept responsibility for becoming HIV-infected (infection between homosexuals)>>, and <<I am not going to be at the mercy of anger due to the infection (harmful effects of medicines, heterosexual)>>.

> *Probably he did not know he was infected with HIV, that he did not pass on the infection with any feelings of malice, and that passing on the infection was not intentional.(#26, female, score: 53)*

The category [Ready to fully live one's own life] encompassed subcategories that described participants' motivation to <<Live while regretting one's behavior that led to infection (homosexual infection)>>, <<I will go straight>>, and to <<Be thoroughly prepared for the onset of AIDS and dying before others>>. Some participants reported that this mental state was not reached immediately after discovering the infection, and was not easy. At the time the infection was discovered, some participants became depressed and desperate. However, having people around them providing support allowed them to organize things in their minds and behave in ways to help discover how to live their life.

> *What happened has happened and there is nothing I can do about it. I can't hide from reality. So, go back to point zero and think about how I want to live my life, that's what I've done. Speaking from experience, having done my best including trying to be mentally positive, I think in the end it's best to live my life honestly and properly. (#34, male, score: 44)*

4. Discussion

4.1. Difficulties experienced by people with HIV

Previous studies have shown that major barriers for people infected with HIV in remaining motivated about re-employment are anxiety about their health, education and skills, and workplace discrimination [23, 24]. Although the present study largely focused on those who were already working, there are a range of difficulties faced by people with HIV in terms of their physical and social condition and self-concept. The experience of having been [Cut off from society because of the name of the illness] was only found in the low SOC group. This suggests they had experienced direct (enacted) stigma, such as <<Being told that my disability was not normal>> or <<Being told that you do not get that disease if you live a normal life>>. Most participants felt that although stigma from the community was unfair, they could not do anything about it and had to accept it. A previous study [25] found that enacted stigma and vicarious stigma (where a person hears of another's experience) were significantly associated with depression and self-stigma. These experiences are likely to damage a person's SOC and prevent its restoration. This was true for the low SOC group in the present study. A study focused on mental illness by Lundberg et al. is the only research to date that has examined the relationship between SOC and stigma [26]. The present study is the first to examine the relationship between the SOC of people with HIV and their experiences of stigma.

Lundberg et al. [26] found the experience of having been socially rejected was significantly associated with low SOC. This association was stronger ($\beta = -0.357$, $p < 0.001$) than for empowerment ($p < 0.02$) or self-esteem ($p < 0.01$). The results of their research, and those of the present study, confirm the close relationship between SOC and stigma. This is a significant finding; however, the ways in which experiences of stigma impact on SOC have not yet been sufficiently investigated.

The present study found that people with HIV experienced direct stigma in medical settings and in the workplace. In particular, two participants who reported experiencing stigma at work were employed under the Disability Act. This suggests that experiencing stigma in medical facilities and workplaces, where a higher level of understanding is usually expected, may result in an unmanageable and incomprehensible situation that causes confusion and a sense of powerlessness. If people working under the Disability Act experience stigma at work, they have lost a place to feel safe, which may result in despair. Furthermore, unlike vicarious stigma, enacted stigma is inescapable, and may result in beliefs such as HIV infection being the reason for stigma. Therefore, stigma may negatively affect SOC, and this may explain why a person decides not to reveal their illness at work or in other situations.

4.2. Coping by people with HIV

Coping strategies of participants with high SOC in the present study were classified as coping with the environments they encountered and cognitive coping. The findings showed that encounters with favorable environments maintained or improved SOC. However, in those who did not report good encounters with people or favorable environments, their high SOC was attributed to cognitive and behavioral coping. Cognitive coping referred to how encountered environments were perceived. Behavioral coping referred to how they changed their own environment. High SOC is considered to make cognitive and behavioral coping possible.

4.2.1. The surrounding environment

Categories extracted relating to the surrounding environment represented experiences of favorable working conditions and workplace cultures, as well as positive human relationships. Previous theoretical [13] and qualitative studies have indicated that there is a significant relationship between working environment and SOC [27]. SOC reflects one's trust toward one's life and the wider context (surrounding people and environment). In SOC theory, "legitimate others" are those who provide this sense of being trusted, loved, watched, and recognized. Legitimate others bring a sense of security and the feeling that one is not alone. They also give people meaning in life, energy, and courage [13].

http://dx.doi.org/10.5772/65775

4.3. High SOC coping strategies

A coping strategy in participants with high SOC concerned the challenge of how they should behave in a situation they could not control (e.g., strong stigma against HIV, a workplace culture that did not allow diversity, difficult work conditions, unstable physical condition, and relationship breakup). These are situations that participants could not do anything about by themselves. Participants in the high SOC group reported trying their best to cope with these stressors.

According to Antonovsky [13], people with high SOC tend to view the world as consistent. An effective way of holding this perspective is flexibly controlling the boundaries of important areas in life. For example, to avoid distress, they might bring part of their lives to a peripheral area that was not as important to them. Participants with high SOC in the present study tried to actively change the boundaries between what was important to them and reality, including compromising on job content and conditions, depending on their own physical condition and environment, and changing the goals of their work or life. They coped with events that had become incomprehensible and unmanageable by bringing them to areas that were less important to them. Kraaij found that people with HIV who were capable of making goal adjustment in their lives were able to maintain positive mental health [28]. The present study confirmed the importance of flexibly adjusting goals.

The group with high SOC escaped from the chaos of their reality by neutrally perceiving the events relating to their infection and by calmly and objectively observing their reality. Antonovsky [13] stated that people with high SOC are not trapped by their emotions too long; instead, they define the nature and dimension of their problems, deal with them, and explore ways to move from chaos to order. The present study found the high SOC group used behavioral coping strategies, deciding to do something about it, taking action, and not allowing themselves to be defeated by a sense of uncertainty or difficulties. Antonovsky [13] regarded participation in consequences as an important element of meaningfulness. Participation in consequences encompasses factors such as autonomy and participation in decision-making; for example, accepting current challenges, taking responsibility, and making decisions as to what to do or not to do. The accumulation of these experiences nurtures a sense of meaningfulness. In the present study, many participants in the low SOC group had given up on having an intimate relationship. In contrast, those in the high SOC group took action and tried not to be defeated by uncertainty or difficulties. Even if the consequence of their action did not turn out as expected, this group considered their judgment to be meaningful because their will and behavior had been reflected in the consequences.

Participants in the high SOC group who were infected through sexual contact tried to accept their responsibility for the infection. In contrast, those in the low SOC group were not able to overcome their sense of being victimized. Antonovsky [13] suggests that many stressors cause problems of blame where responsibility is attributed to others. Those with low SOC tend to blame other people or factors for their problems. In the present study, some participants with high SOC reported experiencing confusion and depression when they learned about their infection or progression to AIDS, despairing and not caring anymore about what they did. However, they reported being able to find ways to cognitively and emotionally cope with their problems, taking responsibility for their infection, placing the infection within an area of life they could control, and viewing their problems objectively. These participants coped with the difficulties of HIV infection by feeling that they were participating in the consequences.

4.4. Suggestions for practice

Although it is not surprising that only those with low SOC reported experiencing direct stigma, it is a reality that should not be ignored. Direct stigma has a serious, negative impact on people with HIV. In the present study, direct stigma was reported by people who were working under the framework of the Disability Act. Even if an employer or a human resources manager has knowledge about HIV infection, other colleagues may not share the same level of understanding. HIV infection is an invisible disability, and those employed under the Disability Act tend to be regarded by others with suspicion. Some participants in the present study reported that they did not know what to say when asked by fellow workers what disease they had. Educating employers, human resource managers, and other staff about HIV through corporate training is urgently needed.

In addition, from an industrial health perspective, it may be necessary to develop workplace cultures in which people with health conditions can work and receive treatment without distress. A workplace in which workers with HIV can feel comfortable will be a good workplace for all employees. Everyone risks losing their health at some point. Therefore, it is important to improve working conditions so employees can work according to their health conditions and lifestyles. However, it is also important that good relationships are developed with managers and colleagues through regular communication, allowing people with HIV to gain trust, and be seen as a reliable working member of society. The present analysis showed that participants' social skills were an important factor for SOC, and although changes are needed in the workplace, people with HIV also need to make their own efforts to fulfill the role of a worker.

The attitudes of those with high SOC make them more likely to cope successfully. This provides important clues for future interventions and education. Although international studies have accumulated a wide knowledge base about interventions for HIV infection [29, 30], there have been few studies in Japan. It is important to increase coping skills to support people with HIV, including suggesting alternative ways of thinking about their situation. Unconditional support from families and significant others is important.

4.5. Limitations

First, no participants in the high SOC group reported experiencing direct stigma. However, this may not mean that they never experienced direct stigma. They may have had experiences they did not report or did not recognize as stigma. Future studies should examine whether or not participants had real experience of stigma, quantitatively clarify how the impact of stigma was recognized, and examine the association between stigma and SOC.

Second, participants in the present study might have been patients in particularly good physical and mental condition. Participants were selected by the nurses working in the specialized medical facilities, and limited to those considered by the nurses to be in a good enough condition to be interviewed. It may be that recruited participants were those who had good relationships with the nurses and who were considered easy to communicate with. The facilities advised that 5–10 patients declined to participate because they came for treatment during working hours and did not have time for an interview or did not feel well. Some of those who were not asked to participate may not have been physically or mentally well, or may not have had a good relationship with their medical professionals. The present study stopped recruiting participants after 40 interviews, as this was deemed the saturation level. However, it is possible that if those who declined had been included, other categories of experiences might have been extracted. Therefore, the interpretation of the present results requires some caution.

Acknowledgements

This study was supported by JSPS KAKENHI Grant Number 24530731.

Author details

Tomoko Omiya*, Yoshihiko Yamazaki, Megumi Shimada, Kazuko Ikeda, Seiko Ishiuchi-Ishitani and Katsumi Ohira

*Address all correspondence to: toomiya-tky@umin.ac.jp

Toho University, Tokyo, Japan

References

[1] AIDS surveillance committee of Ministry of Health, Labour and Welfare. 2010 AIDS outbreak trend annual report in Japan. [Internet]. 2011/05/23 [Updated: 2011/05/23]. Available from: http://api-net.jfap.or.jp/status/2014/14nenpo/h26gaiyo.pdf [Accessed: 2012/06/27.]

[2] Lohse, N., Hansen, A. B. E., Pedersen, G., Kronborg, G., Gerstoft, J., Sorensen, H. T. Survival of persons with and without HIV infection in Denmark, 1995–2005. Annals of Internal Medicine. 2007; **146**(2); 87–95.

[3] Mizushima, D., Oka, S. HIV infection in Japan. Clinical Microbiology. 2010; **37**(6):684–689.

[4] McGurk, S. R., Mueser, K. T., DeRosa, T. J., Wolfe, R. Work, recovery, and comorbidity in schizophrenia: a randomized controlled trial of cognitive remediation. Schizophrenia Bulletin. 2009; **35**(2):319–335.

[5] Swindells, S., Mohr, J., Justis, J. C., Berman, S., Squier, C., Wagener, M. M. Quality of life in patients with human immunodeficiency virus infection: impact of social support, coping style and hopelessness. International Journal of STD & AIDS. 1999; **10**(6):383–91.

[6] Omiya, T., Yamazaki, Y., Shimada, M., Ikeda, K., Ishiuchi-Ishitani, S., Ysuno, Y. S. Mental health of patients with human immunodeficiency virus in Japan: a comparative analysis of employed and unemployed patients. AIDS Care. 2014; **26**(11):1370–1378. DOI: 10.1080/09540121.2014.913765

[7] Brooks, R. A., Klosinski, L. E. Assisting persons living with HIV AIDS to return to work: programmatic steps for AIDS service organizations. AIDS Education and Prevention. 1999; **11**(3):212–223.

[8] Hergenrather, K. C., Rhodes, S. D., Clark, G. The employment perspectives study: identifying factors influencing the job-seeking behavior of persons living with HIV/AIDS. AIDS Education and Prevention. 2005; **17**(2):131–142. DOI: 10.1521/aeap.17.3.131.62905

[9] Medley, A. M., Kennedy, C. E., Lunyolo, S., Sweat, M. D. Disclosure outcomes, coping strategies, and life changes among women living with HIV in Uganda. Qualitative Health Research. 2009; **19**(12):1744–1754. DOI: 10.1177/1049732309353417

[10] Cohen, M., Hoffman, R. G., Cromwell, C., Schmeidler, J., Ebrahim, F., Carrera, G. The prevalence of distress in persons with human immunodeficiency virus infection. Psychosomatics. 2002; **43**(1):10–15.

[11] Fesko, S. L. Workplace experiences of individuals who are HIV plus and individuals with cancer. Rehabilitation Counseling Bulletin. 2001; **45**(1):2–11.

[12] Heckman, T. G., Anderson, E. S., Sikkema, K. J., Kochman, A., Kalichman, S. C., Anderson, T. Emotional distress in nonmetropolitan persons living with HIV disease enrolled in a telephone-delivered, coping improvement group intervention. Health Psychology. 2004; **23**(1):94–100. DOI: 10.1037/0278-6133.23.1.94

[13] Antonovsky, A. Unraveling the Mystery of Health: How People Manage Stress and Stay Well. 1st ed. San Francisco, California: Jossey-Bass Publishers; 1987.

[14] Antonovsky, A. Health, Stress, and Coping: New Perspectives on Mental and Physical Well-Being. San Francisco, California: Jossey-Bass Publishers; 1979.

[15] Eriksson, M., Lindstrom, B. Antonovsky's sense of coherence scale and its relation with quality of life: a systematic review. Journal of Epidermal Community Health. 2007; **61**(11):938–944. DOI: 10.1136/jech.2006.056028

[16] Togari, T., Yamazaki, Y. Examination of the reliability and factor validity of 13-item five-point version sense of coherence scale. Journal of Health and Human Ecology. 2005; **71**(4):168–182.

[17] Lofland, J. Analyzing Social Settings: A Guide to Qualitative Observation and Analysis. 4th ed. Belmont, California: Wadsworth; 2006. pages.

[18] Creswell, J W. Qualitative Inquiry and Research Design: Choosing Among Five Traditions. Thousand Oaks, California: Sage Publications; 2007. pages.

[19] Söderhamn, U., Dale B., Söderhamn, O. Narrated lived experiences of self-care and health among rural-living older persons with a strong sense of coherence. Psychology Research and Behavior Management. 2011; **4**:151–158.

[20] Ahola, A. J., Saraheimo, M., Forsblom, C., Hietala, K., Groop, P. H. The cross-sectional associations between sense of coherence and diabetic microvascular complications, glycaemic control, and patients' conceptions of type 1 diabetes. Health and Quality of Life Outcomes. 2010; **8**:142. DOI: 10.1186/1477-7525-8-142.

[21] Urakawa, K., Yokoyama, K., Itoh, H. Sense of coherence is associated with reduced psychological responses to job stressors among Japanese factory workers. BMC Research Notes. 2012; **5**. DOI: 10.1186/1756-0500-5-247

[22] Ebina, R., Yamazaki, Y. Sense of coherence and coping in adolescents directly affected by the 1991–5 war in Croatia. Promotion & Education. 2008; **15**(4):5–10.

[23] Brooks, R. A., Martin, D. J., Ortiz, D. J., Veniegas, R. C. Perceived barriers to employment among persons living with HIV/AIDS. AIDS Care. 2004; **16**(6):756–766. DOI: 10.1080/09540120412331269594

[24] Martin, D. J, Brooks, R. A., Ortiz, D. J., Veniegas, R. C. Perceived employment barriers and their relation to workforce-entry intent among people with HIV/AIDS. Journal of Occupational Health Psychology. 2003; **8**(3):181–194.

[25] Steward, W. T., Herek, G. M., Ramakrishna, J., Bharat, S., Chandy, S., Wrubel, J. HIV-related stigma: adapting a theoretical framework for use in India. Social Science & Medicine. 2008; **67**(8):1225–1235. DOI: 10.1016/j.socscimed.2008.05.032

[26] Lundberg, B., Hansson, L., Wentz, E., Bjorkman, T. Are stigma experiences among persons with mental illness, related to perceptions of self-esteem, empowerment and sense of coherence? Journal of Psychiatric and Mental Health Nursing. 2009; **16**(6):516–522. DOI: 10.1111/j.1365-2850.2009.01418.x

[27] Feldt, T., Kinnunen, U., Mauno, S. A mediational model of sense of coherence in the work context: a one-year follow-up study. Journal of Organizational Behavior. 2000; **21**(4):461–476.

[28] Kraaij, V., Van der Veek, S. M., Garnefski, N., Schroevers, M., Witlox, R., Maes, S. Coping, goal adjustment, and psychological well-being in HIV-infected men who have sex with men. AIDS Patient Care and STDs. 2008; **22**(5):395–402. DOI: 10.1089/apc.2007.0145

[29] Antoni, M. H., Carrico, A. W., Duran, R. E., Spitzer, S., Penedo, F., Ironson, G. Randomized clinical trial of cognitive behavioral stress management on human immunodeficiency virus viral load in gay men treated with highly active antiretroviral therapy. Psychosomatic Medicine. 2006; **68**(1):143–151. DOI: 10.1097/01.psy.0000195749.60049.63

[30] Carrico, A. W., Antoni, M. H., Pereira, D. B., Fletcher, M. A., Klimas, N., Lechner, S. C. Cognitive behavioral stress management effects on mood, social support, and a marker of antiviral immunity are maintained up to 1 year in HIV-infected gay men. International Journal of Behavioral Medicine. 2005; **12**(4):218–216. DOI: 10.1207/s15327558ijbm1204_2

Chapter 6

The Contextual Environmental Factors Shaping Disclosure of HIV Status across Populations Groups in Sub-Saharan Africa

Sphiwe Madiba

Additional information is available at the end of the chapter

http://dx.doi.org/10.5772/66682

Abstract

Disclosure of HIV-positive status is a public health intervention strategy to reduce HIV infections and improve HIV treatment and care. While disclosure occurs for different reasons for different population groups, the focus of studies has been on programmatic concerns such as disclosure to sexual partners to prevent HIV transmission or to prevent mother to child transmission of HIV. However, HIV disclosure occurs within a broad range of social and cultural contexts. Disclosure is facilitated or deterred by relationships at play within the social context beyond just the need for prevention of HIV. This chapter will highlight how the construction of HIV as an incurable, fatal, and contagious disease, stigma and discrimination, cultural and societal norms, secrecy, and the contextual environment influence HIV disclosure across different population groups. The chapter further demonstrated that stigma is the threat that connects the contextual environment and negatively influences disclosure across different population groups. This chapter is based on disclosure studies conducted in South Africa and extensive findings from disclosure research from sub-Saharan Africa. The data comprise qualitative studies on disclosing HIV to perinatally infected children by caregivers, the parental disclosure of own HIV-positive status to HIV-negative children, disclosure to sexual partners, disclosure to parents, and adolescent self-disclosure to romantic partners and friends.

Keywords: disclosure, stigma, secrecy, people living with HIV, cultural context, Southern Africa

1. Introduction

Disclosure has been an area of concern since the beginning of the HIV epidemic and the focus of research for decades. Extensive research has been done to explore the different types of disclosure, the process of disclosure, and patterns of disclosure. HIV disclosure includes an array of behaviors associated with the practice in which HIV-infected persons disclose their HIV serostatus to their partners, family members, or friends; or when a child is informed of her/his own HIV status [1]. Disclosure of HIV-positive serostatus is an integral component of public health prevention and treatment interventions and has been associated with many potential benefits. To sexual partners, disclosure occurs to enable safer sexual choices, to access prevention of mother to child transmission (PMTCT) of HIV programs, to gain emotional and financial support, and to protect the partner from HIV infection. To family members, disclosure occurs to gain various forms of support such as support for treatment adherence, emotional support, and protecting others from HIV. Lastly, to healthcare workers, disclosure occurs to access treatment and care services [2]. Although it is accepted that disclosure is associated with many beneficial outcomes such as increased social support, improved treatment adherence, decreased experienced stigma, greater well-being, and healthier behaviors. HIV disclosure also carries important risks evident by low disclosure rates among different population groups in sub-Saharan Africa (SSA).

The emphasis of most disclosure studies has been on the individual factors affecting low disclosure rates of the different population groups, while disclosure of HIV-positive serostatus is a complex phenomenon in which social, economic, political, cultural, and environmental aspects are interrelated. Disclosure is complicated by the close and complex relationship between disclosure, stigma, and culture which impacts on each other [3]. Furthermore, HIV disclosure is a complex and difficult personal matter that entails communication about a potentially life threatening, stigmatized, and transmissible infection [4]. The attempt to normalize nondisclosure by people affected by and infected with HIV, makes disclosure even more complex, given that the desire to maintain silence about an HIV test persists in many societies. In fact, there seems to be some level of normalcy when people living with HIV (PLHIV) do not talk about their illness when they anticipate and or experience stigma and discrimination [2, 5]. The normalization of silence is also shaped by the general understanding and evidence that disclosure is not always beneficial, positive, or advantageous to the individual. In fact, it is argued that HIV disclosure carries with it higher levels of risk and vulnerability [6], as the individual who discloses can never predict the response or reaction elicited by the disclosure.

The perception of HIV-related stigma shapes people's concerns about what might happen if they disclose. Consequently, people scan their social environment before they decide whether or not they should disclose their HIV status, and disclosure is deterred if individuals live in communities where HIV stigma is present [7, 8]. Steward et al. [9] argue that PLHIV do not need to encounter actual enactments of stigma to fear its social consequences, but being acutely aware of the potential for stigma or having witnessed stigmatization and discrimination against PLHIV raises the fear of stigma and shape their patterns of disclosure. This fear of stigma leads to people affected and infected by HIV adopting coping strategies such as disclosure avoidance or secrecy and silence to protect self from stigma [10].

A general assumption among researchers and policy makers working in the field of HIV prevention was that the availability of antiretroviral treatment (ART) and the beneficial outcomes of ART would increase the rates of disclosure in SSA. However, the low rates of HIV disclosure are an indication that the availability and increased access to ART in SSA are not changing the underlying structural causes of stigma contributing to the reluctance of people to disclose. Extensive research in SSA indicates that HIV-stigma is continuing to deter disclosure [11, 12]. Research indicates that disclosing one's HIV status carries an extraordinary degree of exposure [5], and that by disclosing, the person no longer struggles with concealing a secret, but may now be exposed to stigma [13]. The reluctance of individuals to disclose their HIV status is despite evidence that taking ART assist PLHIV to return to a healthy state by halting or reversing the progression of the diseases thereby hiding the physical and visible stigmatizing attributes of HIV.

Research suggests that the process of normalizing HIV through ART is socially complex, slow, and uneven in many communities in SSA [5, 14, 15]. Since the wide access to ART has not succeeded in increasing the rates of disclosure, there is a need to revisit how disclosure is conceptualized by individuals infected and affected by HIV in their contextual environments under which disclosure is more or less likely to occur.

2. Research on disclosure across populations

While disclosure occurs for different reasons for different population groups, the focus of studies has been on the reasons for disclosure and nondisclosure for the individuals. The chapter will use empirical data to demonstrate that disclosure is not driven by behavior only but by the contextual environment within which disclosure should occur or occurs. The chapter also uses findings from qualitative research conducted from 2009 to 2013 in South Africa to demonstrate how the construction of HIV, stigma and discrimination, secrecy, cultural norms, and the contextual environment influence HIV disclosure across different population groups [16–21].

The chapter will further demonstrate that the contextual environment is comparable across population groups, and that stigma is a constant factor which influences the social context of all population groups and a key factor in the reluctance of people affected and infected with HIV to disclose.

2.1. Study design and population

This chapter reports on the findings of four qualitative studies. The study design employed for three of the studies was qualitative explorative, and the fourth study used grounded theory design. The study participants included caregivers of perinatally infected children aged 6–13 years, HIV-positive parents of negative children aged 7–18 years, HIV-infected postnatal women in PMTCT program, and perinatally infected adolescents aged 12–18 years.

2.2. Study settings

All the studies were conducted in primary health facilities (PHC) and ART clinics of four hospitals in Mpumalanga and Gauteng provinces, South Africa. The four ART clinics were based in three community hospitals and one tertiary hospital and 34 health facilities providing ART services to adults and children living with HIV through the nurse-initiated and managed antiretroviral treatment initiative. The health facilities in Mpumalanga province were located in the rural subdistricts of Nkangala district, whereas the Gauteng province facilities were located in urban Tshwane district.

2.3. Data collection

The studies used focus group discussions (FGDs) and in-depth interviews (IDIs) to collect data with purposely selected participants for all the studies. The investigators (author as a principal investigator and a coinvestigator), Master of Public Health students and research assistants conducted the interviews. All interviews were conducted in local languages.

2.4. Data analysis

Data from three of the studies were analyzed using thematic analysis of the verbatim transcribed interviews. NVivo version 10, qualitative data analysis software, was used for coding. All the analyses were conducted either by the author or under the direct supervision of the author. The grounded theory study was analyzed by the author using constant comparison analysis.

2.5. Ethics

All the studies received ethical clearance from Medunsa Campus Research and Ethics Committee of the University of Limpopo; the author was affiliated with the institution at the time of the conduct of the studies. Permissions to conduct the studies were obtained from relevant provincial, district, and facility authorities of the two provinces. Written informed consent was obtained from all the participants who could legally consent, and assent was obtained from adolescents who were below 18 years of age. Participation for all the participants was voluntary, and privacy and confidentiality were safeguarded.

3. Disclosing a child's HIV status

A grounded theory study was conducted to explore how a sample of caregivers of children receiving ART view and experience HIV disclosure to perinatal infected children. Nine FGDs were conducted with 52 caregivers of children between 6 and 13 years. Data were collected between November 2009 and March 2010. Four main themes emerged from the data: thoughts of death and dying, the influence of media, fear of discrimination, and secrecy illustrate how the contextual environment is influencing disclosure and nondisclosure to infected children.

Caregivers delayed disclosure to children because they believe that their children would live in fear of death and dying. HIV disclosure to children was also influenced by the fear of stigma that the caregivers perceived to be present in their communities, and they feared that the children would be discriminated, mocked, teased, and socially rejected.

The thing is..., whenever you mention HIV, they know that AIDS kills, so..., when you tell her, she will know that she is going to die. That is what we are afraid of..., because the child will live thinking that she is going to die. Isn't it we hear that AIDS kills..., that when you have AIDS, you die? When you tell the child about it she will think she is dying (37-year-old mother of a 6-year-old).

I am afraid it will be known by everyone in my neighborhood and they will start saying "we don't want to play with this one he is HIV positive; he will infect us" (36-year-old mother of an 11-year-old).

Nondisclosed caregivers maintained silence to protect their children from stigma, discrimination, mockery, and social rejection, while disclosed caregivers kept the child's diagnosis secret from families and neighbors. The fear that the child would not keep the secret but would tell other children at school and in the neighborhood that he/she has HIV and subject the family to stigmatization featured strongly as a reason for delaying disclosure to infected children.

When I told him I said this is your secret because I am afraid of stigma, I told him it's only the family that knows because I see the way other people lack knowledge about this thing [HIV]. I am afraid of rejection (32-year-old mother of a 9-year-old).

We didn't tell him to talk or not to talk, but the way I see it, he does not talk, I wouldn't like him to talk (24-year-old brother of an 8-year-old).

4. Disclosing parental status to children

Focus group interviews were conducted to explore the disclosure of parent's own HIV-positive status to HIV-negative children accessing ART from an academic hospital in South Africa. Six FGDs were conducted between November 2010 and January 2011 with 47 HIV-positive parents of children aged between 7 and 18 years. The data present four main themes fear of death and dying, the influence of media, fear of discrimination, and secrecy to highlight the social context influencing disclosure of parental HIV status to children.

Parental disclosure occurs within an environment where children think that AIDS kills and the thoughts of fear of death and dying characterized the discussions of disclosure of parent's HIV status to children. Parents delayed disclosure because they believed that children believe that AIDS kills and would be concerned that their parents may die too.

Children know that people infected with HIV die, you become afraid to tell because the child will say "my mother is going to die" so you become afraid to tell (Mother of 2 children).

I am scared that he will feel miserable and maybe think my mother is dying, my father is dead, my mother is also going to die..., so who are we going to be left with..., what is going to happen? (Widowed mother of 2 children).

Parents perceived the television and media as negatively influencing children's perceptions of HIV-positive people. They were concerned that media portrays HIV as a debilitating, fatal disease. This created fear for parental disclosure of HIV status to children.

My child watches HIV-related drama on TV, many of these dramas show that a person who is HIV positive end up dying. That thing is the one that makes me afraid to tell my child. That is the reason why I am afraid to tell (Father of 3 children).

Fear of stigma and discrimination was one of the main reasons parents delayed HIV status disclosure to children. They had fears that the child may not be able to keep the parent's HIV status secret and were concerned that the family will be subjected to stigma, discrimination, and isolation.

> *The reason for not telling my child is that I have one child who is 7 years old. It is good and not good to tell taking into consideration the child's age and the stigma surrounding this disease (Mother of 1 child).*

> *My reason for not telling is because a child does not have a secret, we have not accepted this disease as a community. Because my child cannot keep a secret, you are going to see people looking down at me (Father of 1child).*

As a result of stigma and discrimination, parents went to considerable lengths to keep their HIV-positive status secret from their children, family members, and community members. Disclosed parents instructed their children to keep the disclosure secret and even when parents did not give their children instructions not to tell other people, they believed that their children understood the nature of the disease and knew that they would not tell people outside the family.

> *Eish..., you know, this child, if you tell him, he is going to tell his friends that my father is going to die; he is having AIDS (Father of 3 children).*

> *At seventeen, she knows that it is a family secret and then if you tell she will never talk (Single mother of 3 children).*

5. Disclosure to sexual partner

The study used FGDs to explore HIV disclosure to sexual partners and significant family members among HIV-positive postnatal women enrolled in a PMTCT program. FGDs were conducted with 25 women aged between 18 and 40 years between November 2010 and January 2011. Three main themes stigma and rejection, protecting the HIV status, and fear of violence highlight the social context influencing disclosure to sexual partners.

The most common reasons for nondisclosure to family members were fear of social rejection and discrimination. Women were fearful of disclosure because they felt that they will be rejected by their family. They further associated disclosure to sexual partners to the risks of discrimination, abandonment, and rejection.

> *My mother has serious problems with HIV-positive people (27yrs single mother).*

> *After I had tested HIV positive, I asked my husband to get tested too, and he was HIV negative. Since that day he never came back home, he has another woman he is staying with now (43yrs married woman).*

> *I told him that I was pregnant and HIV positive, he was happy that I was pregnant, but the issue of me being HIV positive, he did not take it so well. It was the last time I saw him, he left (31yrs single mother).*

Concealing the HIV status was commonly used as a strategy for protecting self from stigma and rejection. However, participating in PMTCT subjected women to scrutiny and questioning and the women devised strategies to continue hiding their HIV status from partners, families, and the community.

http://dx.doi.org/10.5772/66682

My grandmother asked me why I was not breastfeeding my baby and I told her that I was having problems with my breasts and I cannot breastfeed (30yrs single mother).

With my tablets, immediately after collecting them from the clinic, I empty them into sachets, and I throw away the ARVs bottles so that if somebody finds me drinking my ART medication, they would not know what I am taking (26yrs single mother).

The women who did not disclose their HIV-positive status to their sexual partners found disclosure difficult. They were fearful that their partners would react with violence to the disclosure or accuse them of being responsible for the infection.

The main thing that is worrying me is how he is going to feel when I tell him. I'm scared to tell him because he is one person that will want to tell everybody about my status in his family that I'm the one who gave it [HIV] to him (24yrs single mother).

6. Adolescents onward self-disclosure to others

In-depth interviews were conducted with 37 perinatally infected adolescents between December 2012 and July 2013. The study explored how perinatally infected adolescents experienced living with HIV and examined their perceptions and experiences about disclosure and onward self-disclosure to friends, romantic partners, and others. Three themes reaction to knowing HIV diagnosis, fear of stigma and discrimination, and secrecy illustrate the contextual environment within which adolescents receive disclosure and disclose.

Adolescents experienced both positive and negative effects of disclosure. Some described the disclosure event as extremely shocking and hurtful, and some felt like they were dying. They could not figure out how they could have been infected if they did not engage in sexual activities and expressed ambivalent feelings of self-blame.

When I discovered about my HIV status, I did not feel good at all. You think about a lot of things. You think that you no longer have a life. You feel that people can see that you are HIV positive (Male participant; 17yrs).

I was very shattered, and I asked myself what I did before God that I should be infected with HIV (Male participant; 17yrs).

Adolescents were aware of the secret nature of their HIV diagnosis, and they considered their HIV diagnosis a secret. Fear of being gossiped about and stigmatized was an important consideration for keeping their HIV status secret.

My status is my secret and will remain my secret until I am older. It is a secret; the only people who need to know are your family (Male participation, 17yrs).

You must only tell your family members who will not tell other people outside because others are gossipers and will tell other people that this child is HIV positive (Female participant, 14yrs).

Disclosure to friends resulted in stigmatization for some of the adolescents who felt the need to disclose to friends. The subsequent experience of stigma led to secrecy and emotional trauma for the adolescents.

> *I did not know whom to tell, my mother was always crying, always under stress, and I did not know whom to tell. I told myself that I have to break the silence once and for all, then I told my friends, and they started isolating me (Female participation, 14yrs).*

> *I told my friend, and after I had told him, he told others; whenever I pass them, they bothered me (Male participation; 15yrs).*

Adolescents expressed a strong message that their HIV status was truly their secret and expressed anxiety at how difficult disclosure would be. They also feared that their romantic partners and friends would react in a negative way to disclosure.

> *It will be too painful to me to tell my friends because they will perceive me differently (Female participant; 12yrs).*

> *If I tell him, he will leave me (Female participant; 18yr).*

> *I don't want them judging me, and I am afraid that my best friend will refuse to play with me (Male participation; 14yrs).*

7. Environmental contextual factors shaping disclosure

7.1. Construction of HIV

HIV testing and disclosure are influenced by cultural and social contexts and to a greater extent by the understandings of HIV and AIDS which are grounded in broader understandings of the long-term illness, death, and social danger [4, 22]. From the beginning of the HIV epidemic, HIV was conceptualized as highly stigmatizing, incurable, fatal, contagious, a threat to the life of others, physically degenerative and disfiguring, and associated with a painful or anesthetic death [23]. Many decades after the first cases of HIV and AIDS, people continue to perceive HIV and AIDs as meaning death and dying in many societies in SSA. People perceive AIDS as a deadly disease and often make no distinction between HIV and AIDS. Having HIV and AIDS is associated with being sick and approaching death and often people are afraid to test while HIV-positive people see no reasons for disclosure from the anticipation of severe stigma [5, 22, 24–27].

Earlier arguments about the construction of HIV/AIDS as meaning death and dying came from the knowledge that in African settings where ART was not readily available, HIV infection was a death sentence [28]. It was therefore anticipated that with the advent of ART the context of stigmatization due to fear of imminent death might be changing. However, despite the increased access to ART and the positive outcomes of treatment, people continue to perceive HIV as signaling death and dying. Jürgensen et al. argue that the memories of AIDS are embedded in narratives and experiences of the death of people and have been imprinted in people's minds [24].

The fear of death and dying is also evident in the way HIV is constructed by perinatally infected children. HIV is primarily constructed in relation to a language of sickness even when children are on ART and are relatively healthy. Perinatal infected children, who started ART at an early age, have no experience of life pre-HIV [14]. Therefore, their construction of

HIV is influenced by that of the adults whose context of HIV is that of a debilitating illness. Daniel points out that in the case of children, adults ignore to emphasize the positive health that people on ART enjoy. As a consequence, children associate HIV with illness and weakness and horror stories about the physical appearance of other people living with HIV [14, 29]. While this negative view of HIV might have been instilled by the adults who care for them and the society as a whole, Domek argues that for some of the children the association of AIDS with death and dying is real. As some of the children have been exposed to the devastating effects of HIV and had seen their parents or other significant family members die [30].

The first public health prevention campaigns perpetuated negative perceptions and heightened the fear of HIV/AIDS. The original billboards used in HIV/AIDS awareness campaigns depicted HIV/AIDS as debilitating, frightening, and fatal disease, by focusing on negative images of sick, dying, and disfigured persons. The portrayal of HIV as a grossly disfiguring disease resulted in individuals relating an HIV-positive test to a death sentence [31–33]. Research indicates that people continue to have ambiguous feelings about physical contact with HIV-positive people and that HIV stigma is still unintentionally reinforced by campaigns addressing HIV/AIDS [34].

Given the fact that the levels of HIV/AIDS-related knowledge are often inversely correlated with stigma [35], it was anticipated that providing people with factual information about HIV/AIDS would lead to stigma reduction in high HIV prevalence settings [36]. However, stigma lingers on; current research from the Democratic Republic of the Congo shows that the fear of HIV/AIDS prompted people to avoid and stigmatize PLHIV through the use of derogatory labels used to portray PLHIV. Labels commonly used, described PLHIV as walking corpses, dangers to others, or people deserving to die before others get infected. Being labeled made PLHIV suffer in silence and afraid to disclose their status [37].

7.2. Contextual environment

HIV disclosure occurs within a broad range of social and cultural contexts that influence the way individuals infected with HIV and affected by HIV perceive risks, the way they make decisions to take or not to take an HIV test, and the way disclosure takes place [4]. The contextual environment comprises the setting and potential contextual factors under which disclosure is more or less likely to occur. HIV-positive individuals, their families, communities, and their sociocultural and political norms constitute this environment [38]. Bailey and Darak refer to the contextual environment as spaces of disclosure and discrimination and point out that disclosure is influenced by spaces of disclosure which ranges from the clinic or hospital, spouses, family members, relatives, and others [39]. While Hardon et al. identified five social spaces that are considered to shape disclosure practices which include international recommendations, household and family settings, couple relationships, parental relationships, and patient-health worker relationships [40]. According to Bailey and Darak [39], these spaces of disclosure are also spaces of discrimination.

Being able to disclose safely within one space or social environment has been shown to increase disclosure rates and enable people to manage HIV stigma [2, 41]. However, the social contexts influence disclosure in a positive and negative way, and the social relations and family dynamics within the spaces of disclosure play a fundamental role in the decision individuals take to disclose or not disclose. Extensive research shows that stigma is often perpetrated within the family and interpersonal space of marriage. Women, in particular, face unique barriers when disclosing within the marital relationship or to sexual partners in the context of high levels of HIV stigma [36, 42–44]. In many settings in the SSA, the risk of being discriminated and rejected is higher on women because more women get tested for HIV and the burden of disclosing is often on them [45].

The importance of and role of cultural context in the practice of HIV disclosure has been reported upon extensively in research. Cultural values affect decisions on HIV disclosure and different cultural contexts shape the disclosure patterns of individuals, families, and communities [1, 43, 46]. HIV is a socially unacceptable disease and results in the community discriminating against an individual who is perceived to have been infected through their lifestyle and personal behavior [6, 47]. HIV is associated with morally disapproved behavior, and contracting HIV is viewed as the responsibility of the individual, exposing people to blame and judgment [23]. Cultural norms continue to play a significant role in the blame-related stigma and shame associated with HIV/AIDS in many communities in SSA [10, 48]. Community beliefs and societal norms also perpetuate gender inequality, further influencing the social, cultural, and personal spaces for disclosure for women. These shared norms influence a woman's decision regarding HIV disclosure thus shaping HIV and disclosure communication within interpersonal space of marriage and intimate relationships [49].

HIV disclosure to infected children is influenced to a greater extent by the cultural and social contexts in the community [4, 38]. The context of disclosure of HIV status to perinatally infected children is fraught with complexities that relate to the social, familial, and cultural environment of the child in which caregivers are reluctant to discuss the diagnosis with their HIV-infected child [50, 51]. It is argued that parental HIV disclosure to children cannot be expected under circumstances where most PLHIV find it hard to disclose to significant adults such as spouse or partners and family members [52].

7.3. Stigma and HIV

Stigma has been a component of HIV/AIDS since the onset of the pandemic. Stigma compromises AIDS responses and is increasingly regarded as one of the key drivers of the spread of HIV in sub-Saharan Africa. The perception of stigma or the fear of the consequences of stigma prevents people from adopting preventive behavior, getting tested, disclosing their serostatus, accessing treatment and care, and adherence to medication [24, 33, 36, 53]. Alonzo and Reynolds defined stigma as"a powerful discrediting and tainting social label that radically changes the way individuals view themselves and are viewed as persons" [23]. The definition by Parker and Aggleton, describe stigma and stigmatization as being shaped by structures of power and culture and a result of the consequences of collective action by groups rather than that of individual behavior [53]. While HIV stigma is defined as socially shared knowledge about the devalued status of PLHIV [9].

Since HIV is a socially unacceptable disease, it is a highly stigmatized condition compared to many other chronic conditions. HIV stigmatization is not only driven by the physical and visible attributes of an HIV-positive person but by social and cultural processes rooted in communities [27, 47, 54]. HIV stigmatization can include avoidance, exclusion, rejection, isolation, violence, service denial, physical distance, awkward social interaction, and blaming [55]. Nonetheless, the fear of gossip is pronounced as a primary form of HIV stigma throughout SSA [5].

7.4. Stigma and disclosure

HIV stigma affects and is affected by HIV disclosure, while high stigma levels severely hamper disclosure rates and results in silence and secrecy [45], disclosure can lead to stigmatization. Stigmatization is considered a significant barrier to HIV disclosure because HIV disclosure may be deterred if individuals live in communities where HIV stigma is present. The fear of stigma discourages disclosure because PLHIV are more likely to disclose in low-stigma contexts where they expect fewer negative consequences [6, 7, 43, 56].

7.5. Stigma, ART and disclosure

The increasing availability of ART in high prevalence settings did not necessarily reduce stigma and discrimination as anticipated. Extensive research indicates that stigma persists among people on ART and significantly impacts their ability to access treatment and disclose their HIV serostatus [12, 15, 24]. Earlier research on HIV stigma assumed that the increased uptake of ART in many settings in sub-Saharan Africa would reduce some of the stigmatizing characteristics of HIV as disease progression is halted or reversed and PLHIV look healthy. To a lesser extent, ART has made it easier for people to disclose to a closed network particularly within the family setting [5]. However, people still fear, anticipate, and experience stigma from others because ART has not been able to change the underlying causes of stigma, particularly, the moral discourses that judge and blame women and men for contracting HIV [12]. Concerns and fear of being stigmatized are also enduring because HIV stigmatization is not only driven by the physical and visible attributes of an HIV-positive person but also by the underlying structural causes of stigma which ART cannot eliminate [52].

Structural stigma refers to the ways in which societal ideologies and institutions perpetuate or exacerbate a stigmatized status [12]. While structural discrimination relates to accumulated institutional practices that work to the disadvantage of stigmatized groups and can operate in the absence of individual prejudice and discrimination [57]. Research suggests that stigma may be increasing at the individual level for people on ART. It is argued that attending an HIV clinic and adhering to ART medication draw attention to HIV-positive people, making their HIV-positive status visible because of taking ART and regular clinical visits and increase HIV stigma [15, 58].

7.6. Secrecy and silence

Secrecy and silence have characterized the HIV/AIDS epidemic in many societies in sub-Saharan Africa. The perceptions of HIV as a stigmatizing and deadly and contagious disease and the fear of stigma often compels PLWHI people affected by HIV to adopt secrecy and silence as a strategy to manage the HIV stigma [5, 10, 12, 25]. Secrecy is defined as any action taken to attempt to conceal the distinguishing marks that would categorize one in a stigmatized group [59, 60]. In the case of HIV, PLHIV conceal HIV-positive status, clinical signs, ongoing treatment, and visits to the treatment center [61].

Secrecy may be used as a strategic tactic to avoid losing control to others as to how they view one [62]. In these situations, silence is used as a strategy of protecting self and to live as normal a life as possible in social contexts where disclosure would have adverse outcomes [26]. Though the focus of research on the use of silence as a strategy is on individuals, Cohen [63] refers to cultural silence as a strategy that is adopted by the whole community or society. One of the reasons for silence at the cultural level is that the group or the community keeps silent about matters which are based on deep-seated cultural taboos whose open discussion would threaten its self-image. Cultural silence explains the normalization of secrecy and silence around the HIV status among population groups across societies.

Secrecy and silence are also used by caregivers of perinatally infected children to protect the children from discrimination [50, 51, 64]. In SSA, culture is also used to explain silence, particularly in the case of children. Adults use cultural silence as an excuse not to communicate to children by saying that "in our culture, we don't talk to children about death they are too young to understand" [29]. The same argument is used to conceal the HIV diagnosis to perinatally infected children by saying the child is too young to know and understand HIV. As a consequence of the secret nature of HIV and the wide acceptance and adoption of cultural silence, children infected with HIV mimic the behavior of the adults around them. Research has shown that children conceal their HIV diagnosis from friends and people outside of their family network as they have seen their caregivers do and as their caregivers have taught them [29, 41, 65].

However, the use of silence or secrecy as a coping strategy has disadvantages; it can be expensive forcing PLHIV to travel far to access ART. It can also reinforce stigma by not challenging it and fuel gossip and blame. Furthermore, silence can inhibit potential social support, compel PLHIV to conceal medicines, and can lead to death and continued HIV transmission [2, 5, 66, 67]. In the case of children affected by HIV, silence undermines their competence, self-worth, confidence, self-esteem, and increases their anxieties [41].

8. Conclusion

The four case studies highlight that undeniably, disclosure of HIV status across different population groups occurs within the social contexts of thoughts of death and dying, the influence of television, unjust discrimination, and a need for secrecy and silence. Within these contexts, individuals manage the disclosure in such a way as to attempt to keep the situation as normal as possible.

The construction of HIV as signaling a death sentence influence disclosing the child's HIV-positive status, disclosing parental status to HIV-negative children, and disclosing HIV-positive status to family, particularly to elderly parents. The fear of death and dying remains a barrier for caregivers who continue to delay disclosure to perinatally infected children and

http://dx.doi.org/10.5772/66682

parental self-disclosure of HIV-positive status to HIV-negative children. The fear of death and dying is intricately linked to the fear-based messaging used on TV campaigns designed to create HIV/AIDS awareness in South Africa. When HIV is perceived as meaning death and dying, disclosure is delayed despite parents and children receiving ART for an extended duration of time and experiencing the positive gains of ART medication.

The construction of HIV as death and dying also influenced the perceptions of perinatally infected adolescents about disclosure significantly. Perinatally infected adolescents experienced receiving disclosure of their HIV diagnosis as painful and traumatic and described their HIV diagnosis as a death sentence.

Fear of death and dying also deterred postnatal women from disclosing their HIV-positive status to their elderly parents. They also described their HIV diagnosis as a death sentence and perceived their parents as too old and frail to deal with the death sentence that their child had just received.

HIV disclosure across the different population groups was surrounded by secrecy and silence. Secrecy was used to a larger extent by caregivers of perinatally infected children and HIV-positive parents to protect children from harmful emotional consequences of disclosure such as fear of death and dying and stigma and discrimination. Postnatal HIV-positive women also used secrecy to protect their HIV status from their family member, partners, and the community as a whole. Caregivers of perinatally infected children, HIV-positive parents, and HIV-positive postnatal women devoted considerable energy to manipulate their social and contextual environments to conceal the HIV status for as long as possible. They commonly substituted HIV for socially accepted diseases and used false names to describe their illness, used various strategies to hide ART medication, or rescheduled the time for taking ART medication.

Perinatally infected children subsequently mimic the behavior of the adult caregivers around them and also conceal their HIV diagnosis. Perinatally infected adolescents argue that their HIV status is their secret and maintained secrecy to be accepted by their peers but also to protect themselves from stigma and isolation. The fear of HIV-related stigma compels HIV infected and affected individuals to adopt coping strategies of secrecy and silence to protect self and or family from stigma and discrimination. Secrecy is viewed as an effective strategy for maintaining a normal life and has been greatly normalized in society.

Stigma and discrimination were a constant barrier for disclosure to sexual partners, family members, perinatally infected children, HIV-negative children, and romantic partners. Since HIV disclosure takes on different meanings for different population groups even within similar contextual environments, the fear of the different manifestation of stigma is experienced differently by population groups. Stigma was more pronounced for disclosing HIV status to infected children and during parental self-disclosure of HIV-positive status to children. The fear of stigma was also a key consideration for nondisclosure to romantic partners and friends by perinatally infected adolescents. Stigma is such a powerful barrier to disclosure such that even when individuals affected and infected with HIV do not experience enactments of stigma, being aware of the potential for stigma in their contextual environments shapes their disclosure pattern.

Given that disclosure of HIV status to perinatally infected children is more complex than that of adults, it is imperative that disclosure of HIV status to others by HIV-positive adults is understood because the social and cultural contexts of the adults providing care to perinatally infected children shapes the disclosure to children. As a result, self-disclosure to romantic partners by perinatally infected adolescents is as complex as that of disclosure among adults because their contextual environment is shaped by that of the adults too. The complexity of disclosure to perinatally infected children is aggravated by the fact that they may experience two aspects of disclosure; first, when they receive disclosure about their HIV-positive status and second when they receive their parental HIV-positive status. Both disclosure occurrences are saddled with sociocultural challenges affecting disclosure to adults within the communities.

A clear understanding of the contextual environment where disclosure occurs should inform interventions to create enabling environments for safe disclosure for the different population groups. It is imperative that the extent and effect of stigma and discrimination should not be underestimated or ignored by healthcare workers and other key stakeholders such as policy makers who have a vital role to play in reducing stigma. The challenge for researchers is to explore how HIV-related stigma could be overcome to enable people to disclose safely within their spaces or contextual environments. The understanding of the contextual environment or the spaces where disclosure and discrimination occurs will greatly influence the development of interventions to address stigma as being influenced by structural factors beyond behavior.

Author details

Sphiwe Madiba

Address all correspondence to: Sphiwe_madiba@embanet.com

School of Public Health, Faculty of Health Sciences, Sefako Makgatho Health Sciences University, Pretoria, South Africa

References

[1] Qiao S, Li X, Stanton B. Disclosure of parental HIV infection to children: a systematic review of global literature. AIDS & Behavior. 2013;17(1):369–89.

[2] Greeff M, Phetlhu R, Makoae LN, Dlamini PS, Holzemer WL, Naidoo JR, et al. Disclosure of HIV status: experiences and perceptions of persons living with HIV/AIDS and nurses involved in their care in Africa. Qualitative Health Research. 2008;18(3):311–24.

[3] Greeff M. Disclosure and stigma: A cultural perspective. In Stigma, discrimination and living with HIV/AIDS, Springer Netherlands; 2013. pp. 71–95.

[4] Lugalla J, Yoder S, Sigalla H, Madihi C. Social context of disclosing HIV test results in Tanzania. Culture, Health & Sexuality. 2012;14(suppl. 1):S53–66.

[5] Bond VA. It is not an easy decision on HIV, especially in Zambia: opting for silence, limited disclosure and implicit understanding to retain a wider identity. AIDS Care. 2010;22(suppl. 1):6–13.

[6] Chaudoir SR, Fisher JD, Simoni JM. Understanding HIV disclosure: a review and application of the disclosure processes model. Social Science & Medicine. 2011;72(10):1618–29.

[7] Wouters E, van Loon F, van Rensburg D, Meulemans H. Community support and disclosure of HIV serostatus to family members by public-sector antiretroviral treatment patients in the Free State Province of South Africa. AIDS Patient Care and STDs. 2009;23(5):357–64.

[8] Derlega VJ, Winstead BA, Greene K, Serovich J, Elwood WN. Reasons for HIV disclosure/nondisclosure in close relationships: testing a model of HIV–disclosure decision making. Journal of Social & Clinical Psychology. 2004;23(6):747–67.

[9] Steward WT, Herek GM, Ramakrishna J, Bharat S, Chandy S, Wrubel J, et al. HIV-related stigma: adapting a theoretical framework for use in India. Social Science & Medicine. 2008;67(8):1225–35.

[10] Roura M, Urassa M, Busza J, Mbata D, Wringe A, Zaba B. Scaling up stigma? The effects of antiretroviral roll-out on stigma and HIV testing. Early evidence from rural Tanzania. Sexually Transmitted Infections. 2009;85(4):308–12.

[11] Mbonye M, Nakamanya S, Birungi J, King R, Seeley J, Jaffar S. Stigma trajectories among people living with HIV (PLHIV) embarking on a life time journey with antiretroviral drugs in Jinja, Uganda. BMC Public Health. 2013;13(1):804.

[12] Russell S, Zalwango F, Namukwaya S, Katongole J, Muhumuza R, Nalugya R, et al. Antiretroviral therapy and changing patterns of HIV stigmatisation in Entebbe, Uganda. Sociology of Health & Illness. 2016;38(1):58–72.

[13] Smith R, Rossetto K, Peterson BL. A meta-analysis of disclosure of one's HIV-positive status, stigma and social support. AIDS Care. 2008;20(10):1266–75.

[14] Bernays S, Seeley J, Rhodes T, Mupambireyi Z. What am I 'living'with? Growing up with HIV in Uganda and Zimbabwe. Sociology of Health & Illness. 2015;37(2):270–83.

[15] Gilbert L, Walker L. My biggest fear was that people would reject me once they knew my status: stigma as experienced by patients in an HIV/AIDS clinic in Johannesburg, South Africa. Health & Social Care in the Community. 2010;18(2):139–46.

[16] Madiba S. Disclosing HIV to infected children in South Africa in the era of HAART: a grounded theory study on the process, reasons and outcomes of disclosure. World Journal of AIDS. 2012; 2(4):319–29.

[17] Madiba S. The impact of fear, secrecy, and stigma on parental disclosure of HIV status to children: a qualitative exploration with HIV positive parents attending an ART clinic in South Africa. Global Journal of Health Science. 2013;5(2):49.

[18] Madiba S, Letsoalo R. HIV disclosure to partners and family among women enrolled in prevention of mother to child transmission of HIV program: implications for infant feeding in poor resourced communities in South Africa. Global Journal of Health Science. 2013;5(4):1.

[19] Madiba S, Matlala C. Disclosure of parental HIV positive status: what, why, when, and how parents tell their children in the era of HAART in South Africa. World Journal of AIDS. 2012;2(03):194.

[20] Madiba S, Mokgatle M. Perceptions and experiences about self-disclosure of HIV Status among adolescents with perinatal acquired HIV in poor-resourced communities in South Africa. AIDS Research and Treatment. 2016;2016:10.

[21] Madiba S, Mokwena K. Caregivers' barriers to disclosing the HIV diagnosis to infected children on antiretroviral therapy in a resource-limited district in South Africa: a grounded theory study. AIDS Research and Treatment. 2012;2012:10.

[22] de Klerk J. The compassion of concealment: silence between older caregivers and dying patients in the AIDS era, northwest Tanzania. Culture, Health & Sexuality. 2012;14(suppl. 1): S27–38.

[23] Alonzo AA, Reynolds NR. Stigma, HIV and AIDS: an exploration and elaboration of a stigma trajectory. Social Science & Medicine. 1995;41(3):303–15.

[24] Jürgensen M, Tuba M, Fylkesnes K, Blystad A. The burden of knowing: balancing benefits and barriers in HIV testing decisions. a qualitative study from Zambia. BMC Health Services Research. 2012;12(1):1.

[25] Mfecane S. Narratives of HIV disclosure and masculinity in a South African village. Culture, Health & Sexuality. 2012;14(suppl. 1):S109–21.

[26] Moyer E. Faidha gani? What's the point: HIV and the logics of (non)-disclosure among young activists in Zanzibar. Culture, Health & Sexuality. 2012;14(suppl. 1):S67–79.

[27] Visser MJ, Makin JD, Vandormael A, Sikkema KJ, Forsyth BW. HIV/AIDS stigma in a South African community. AIDS Care. 2009;21(2):197–206.

[28] Moore A, Kalanzi DN, Amey FK. To disclose or not to disclose? Lower class parents living with HIV/AIDS in Lomé, Togo. International Journal of Sociology & Social Policy. 2008;28(9/10):351–64.

[29] Daniel M. Keeping the secret: how HIV-positive children in Iringa, Tanzania, respond to the perceived need for silence and secrecy. Journal of Child & Adolescent Mental Health. 2015;27(1):11–23.

[30] Domek GJ. Debunking common barriers to pediatric HIV disclosure. Journal of Tropical Pediatrics. 2010;56(6):440–2.

[31] Liamputtong P, Haritavorn N, Kiatying-Angsulee N. HIV and AIDS, stigma and AIDS support groups: perspectives from women living with HIV and AIDS in central Thailand. Social Science & Medicine. 2009;69(6):862–8.

[32] Lyttleton C. Fleeing the fire: transformation and gendered belonging in Thai HIV/AIDS support groups. Medical Anthropology. 2004;23(1):1–40.

[33] Ogden J, Nyblade L. Common at its core: HIV-related stigma across contexts. Washington, DC: International Center for Research on Women (ICRW); 2005.

[34] Gausset Q, Mogensen HO, Yameogo WME, Berthé A, Konaté B. The ambivalence of stigma and the double-edged sword of HIV/AIDS intervention in Burkina Faso. Social Science & Medicine. 2012;74(7):1037–44.

[35] Kalichman SC, Simbayi LC, Jooste S, Toefy Y, Cain D, Cherry C, et al. Development of a brief scale to measure AIDS-related stigma in South Africa. AIDS & Behavior. 2005;9(2):135–43.

[36] Campbell C, Nair Y, Maimane S, Nicholson J. 'Dying twice': a multi-level model of the roots of AIDS stigma in two South African communities. Journal of Health Psychology. 2007;12(3):403–16.

[37] Mupenda B, Duvall S, Maman S, Pettifor A, Holub C, Taylor E, et al. Terms used for people living with HIV in the Democratic Republic of the Congo. Qualitative Health Research. 2014;24(2):209–16.

[38] Eustace RW, Ilagan PR. HIV disclosure among HIV positive individuals: a concept analysis. Journal of Advanced Nursing. 2010;66(9):2094–103.

[39] Bailey A, Darak S. Spaces of disclosure and discrimination: case studies from India. In Stigma, discrimination and living with HIV/AIDS: Springer Netherlands; 2013. pp. 229–45.

[40] Hardon A, Desclaux A, Lugalla J. Disclosure in times of ART: a relational analysis of social practices. SAHARA-J: Journal of Social Aspects of HIV/AIDS. 2013;10(suppl. 1):S1–4.

[41] Daniel M, Malinga Apila H, Bj⊘rgo R, Therese Lie G. Breaching cultural silence: enhancing resilience among Ugandan orphans. African Journal of AIDS Research. 2007;6(2):109–20.

[42] Bott S, Obermeyer CM. The social and gender context of HIV disclosure in sub-Saharan Africa: a review of policies and practices. SAHARA-J: Journal of Social Aspects of HIV/AIDS. 2013;10(suppl. 1):S5–16.

[43] Obermeyer CM, Baijal P, Pegurri E. Facilitating HIV disclosure across diverse settings: a review. American Journal of Public Health. 2011;101(6):1011–23.

[44] Madiba S, Letsoalo B. Disclosure to sexual partner and associated factors among HIV positive adult clinic attendees in Johannesburg, South Africa: perspectives of HIV and AIDS across populations. African Journal for Physical Health Education, Recreation and Dance, Supplement 21. 2015;21:100–11.

[45] Klopper C, Stellenberg E, Van der Merwe A. Stigma and HIV disclosure in the Cape Metropolitan area, South Africa. African Journal of AIDS Research. 2014;13(1):37–43.

[46] Kalichman SC, Simbayi LC. HIV testing attitudes, AIDS stigma, and voluntary HIV counselling and testing in a black township in Cape Town, South Africa. Sexually Transmitted Infections. 2003;79(6):442–7.

[47] Simbayi LC, Kalichman S, Strebel A, Cloete A, Henda N, Mqeketo A. Internalized stigma, discrimination, and depression among men and women living with HIV/AIDS in Cape Town, South Africa. Social Science & Medicine. 2007;64(9):1823–31.

[48] Leclerc-Madlala S. Demonising women in the era of AIDS: On the relationship between cultural constructions of both HIV/AIDS and femininity. Society in Transition. 2001;32(1):38–46.

[49] Ojikutu BO, Pathak S, Srithanaviboonchai K, Limbada M, Friedman R, Li S, et al. Community cultural norms, stigma and disclosure to sexual partners among women living with HIV in Thailand, Brazil and Zambia (HPTN 063). PloS One. 2016;11(5):e0153600.

[50] Lesch A, Swartz L, Kagee A, Moodley K, Kafaar Z, Myer L, et al. Paediatric HIV/AIDS disclosure: towards a developmental and process-oriented approach. AIDS Care. 2007;19(6):811–6.

[51] Mahloko JM, Madiba S. Disclosing HIV diagnosis to children in Odi district, South Africa: reasons for disclosure and non-disclosure. African Journal of Primary Health Care & Family Medicine. 2012;4(1):345.

[52] Tiendrebeogo G, Hejoaka F, Belem EM, Compaoré PLG, Wolmarans L, Soubeiga A, et al. Parental HIV disclosure in Burkina Faso: experiences and challenges in the era of HAART. SAHARA-J: Journal of Social Aspects of HIV/AIDS. 2013;10(suppl. 1): S46–59.

[53] Parker R, Aggleton P. HIV and AIDS-related stigma and discrimination: a conceptual framework and implications for action. Social Science & Medicine. 2003;57(1):13–24.

[54] Herek GM. Hate crimes and stigma-related experiences among sexual minority adults in the United States prevalence estimates from a national probability sample. Journal of Interpersonal Violence. 2009;24(1):54–74.

[55] Lyimo RA, Stutterheim SE, Hospers HJ, de Glee T, van der Ven A, de Bruin M. Stigma, disclosure, coping, and medication adherence among people living with HIV/AIDS in Northern Tanzania. AIDS Patient Care and STDs. 2014;28(2):98–105.

[56] Nyblade LC. Measuring HIV stigma: existing knowledge and gaps. Psychology, Health & Medicine. 2006;11(3):335–45.

[57] Link BG, Phelan JC. Conceptualizing stigma. Annual Review of Sociology. 2001;27:363–85.

[58] Makoae LN, Portillo CJ, Uys LR, Dlamini PS, Greeff M, Chirwa M, et al. The impact of taking or not taking ARVs on HIV stigma as reported by persons living with HIV infection in five African countries. AIDS Care. 2009;21(11):1357–62.

[59] Goffman E. Stigma: Notes on a spoiled identity. Jenkins, JH & Carpenter. 1963.

[60] Herek GM, Capitanio JP, Widaman KF. HIV-related stigma and knowledge in the United States: prevalence and trends, 1991–1999. American Journal of Public Health. 2002;92(3):371–7.

[61] Hardon AP, Akurut D, Comoro C, Ekezie C, Irunde HF, Gerrits T, et al. Hunger, waiting time and transport costs: time to confront challenges to ART adherence in Africa. AIDS Care. 2007;19(5):658–65.

[62] Goffman E. Stigma: Notes on the management of a spoiled identity. New York: Simon & Schuster.

[63] Cohen R. Living and teaching across cultures. International Studies Perspectives. 2001;2(2):151–60.

[64] Oberdorfer P, Puthanakit T, Louthrenoo O, Charnsil C, Sirisanthana V, Sirisanthana T. Disclosure of HIV/AIDS diagnosis to HIV-infected children in Thailand. Journal of Paediatrics & Child Health. 2006;42(5):283–8.

[65] Hejoaka F. Care and secrecy: being a mother of children living with HIV in Burkina Faso. Social Science & Medicine. 2009;69(6):869–76.

[66] George MS, Lambert H. 'I am doing fine only because I have not told anyone': the necessity of concealment in the lives of people living with HIV in India. Culture, Health & Sexuality. 2015;17(8):933–46.

[67] Madiba S, Canti-Sigaqa V. Barriers to participate in support groups for people living with HIV: a qualitative study with men receiving antiretroviral treatment in a HIV clinic in Mthatha, South Africa. Global Journal of Health Science. 2012;4(6):119.

Chapter 7

The Persistence of Stigma Linked with HIV/AIDS in Health-Care Contexts: A Chronic Social Incapacity

Oscar Labra and Daniel Thomas

Additional information is available at the end of the chapter

http://dx.doi.org/10.5772/66654

Abstract

The article presents an analysis of the stigmatization of people living with HIV/AIDS (PLHIV/AIDS) within health-care contexts. An overview of the short history of HIV/AIDS and of relevant literature reveals the extent and persistence of the stigmatization of PLHIV/AIDS through a variety of practices and attitudes among health personnel; various public policies have, however, produced a number of measures aimed at alleviating the stigma. The article proposes elements of analysis through which to examine stigma as it is present within the implementation of HIV/AIDS care: knowledge about nature and forms of stigmatization and consequences of practices on health services for PLHIV/AIDS.

Keywords: AIDS/HIV, PLHIV/AIDS, Stigma, Discrimination, health care, medical policy

1. Introduction

Stigma associated with various aspects of HIV/AIDS represents an important challenge for those attempting to mitigate the effects of the pandemic. As a social representation of collective fears surrounding HIV/AIDS and judgment of certain behaviors, this stigma forms a barrier that hinders access to health care and social services for many people living with HIV (PLHIV)/AIDS around the world. Indeed, "the history of illness – and epidemics in particular – is not solely one of viral spread and medical response: it is also a history of suspicion towards [PLHIV/AIDS], avoidance and exclusion" [1]. The relationship between health personnel and PLHIV-AIDS began to change after the outbreak of the pandemic, as has been noted also with reference to cancer and tuberculosis. Several studies [2, 3] have shown that caregiver-patient relationships are significantly affected by social representations of the pandemic. Since the emergence of the pandemic, a significant proportion of the literature has studied the experience of stigma in such contexts as education [4], the family [5, 6], and health care [7–11]. Access to care for PLHIV/AIDS has been affected by discriminatory attitudes toward such dimensions as sexual practices, sexually transmitted infections, homosexuality, prostitution, and the use of hard drugs; indeed, HIV/AIDS was at one time known as the 4H disease (i.e., affecting heroin users, homosexuals, Haitians, and hemophiliacs) [12]. The scope of the pandemic, the medical challenges it presents, and the upheaval it causes in the lives of the infected are all factors contributing to set sufferers apart as a distinct social category. Thus, just as has been noted for handicapped individuals [13], cancer sufferers [14], and tuberculosis victims [15], a particular social significance is associated with PLHIV/AIDS.

It is essential to note that three major stages in the emergence of HIV-AIDS in the public consciousness during the 1980s were determinant for the development of negative (and potentially stigmatizing) significations. The first stage was that of an emerging crisis, approximately covering the years 1981–1982. This stage was characterized by growing fears within the male homosexual population, in particular in New York, Los Angeles, and San Francisco, where that population was especially sizeable, but also among Haitian communities in the United States, as well as heroin addicts and hemophiliacs [16]. In the three metropolitan areas mentioned, physicians at the time noted that the infection seemed to affect previously healthy men who had a known history of homosexuality. At the same time, exploratory medical research began attempts to define the epidemiological characteristics and implications of the new phenomenon. The mass media for its part reported on the disease under headlines such as "Mysterious new ill infects homosexual men and drug addicts" and "The gay plague" [17] as well as referring to the acronym GRID (gay-related immune disease) [12]. The terminology used to describe the symptoms underwent several permutations, notably including "the gay cancer," before the acronym AIDS was more widely adopted in 1982.

The second stage, covering the period 1982–1985, was that of moral panic. The marginality of those affected by the disease and its identification as a "gay plague" were major factors shaping social representations during this period. Characterized by the rapid escalation of alarmist reporting in the media and a growing hysteria surrounding AIDS in the broader population, this stage also coincided with the rise to prominence in the US of the New Right and Moral Majority movements as conservative social forces, whose discourses notably linked AIDS with notions of moral decline and divine judgment.

The third stage, which unfolded during the period 1985–1989, may be termed the management crisis stage, which resulted from a congruence of factors, of which the most publicized was the infection and death of actor Rock Hudson, which had a dramatic impact on the public at large. Overall, this period saw the deepening of the AIDS health-care crisis, as HIV infection, the scope of the spread of AIDS, and its costs for society became more widely understood.

By the 1990s, researchers noted that in the first years of the emergence of HIV/AIDS, health care had been characterized by conspicuous stigmatization and high levels of fear in relation to providing care to PLHIV/AIDS [18–23]. Stigma-inducing behaviors thus appeared very early in the history of PLHIV/AIDS health care needs and, since then, the caregiver-patient relationship has progressively become of greater concern to the research community investigating various aspects of the pandemic.

On examining the 30-year history of the spread of the disease, it is clear that relations between health-care personnel and PLHIV-AIDS have undergone various changes. Yet, as studies have shown, people with HIV/AIDS continue to face stigmatization and discrimination in various facets of their lives [24, 25]. This stigmatization and discrimination, moreover, increase health risks for individuals who already face various other forms of discrimination that hinder their access to HIV tests and health-care services [26]. Other studies, in addition, suggest that stigmatization and discrimination tend to isolate the infected, compromise social support, raise anxiety levels, increase social risks linked with the disclosure of their HIV-positive status, impair housing and employment security, and give rise to obstacles along the health-care continuum [27–29].

2. Conceptualizing stigma

The literature produced in the first two decades of the pandemic did not develop an explicit conceptual basis for a definition stigma that would articulate a nuanced understanding of the phenomenon, referring rather to standard definitions ("mark of disgrace associated with a particular circumstance, quality, or person") or related concepts, such as stereotyping and rejection (e.g., "a distance in the social scale"). Yet even a dictionary, sufficiently perused, tells us that the concept of stigma connotes with manifestations that indicate the presence of something beyond view, superficial signs of a concealed phenomenon [30].

In seeking to define stigma more precisely, many authors cite the conceptualization proposed by Goffman (1963) in Notes on the Management of Spoiled Identity, a work that has engendered many subsequent inquiries into the nature, sources, and consequences of stigma. In ancient Greece, the word stigma designated physical marks "designed to expose something unusual and bad about [the bearer's] moral status [13]." As a social and cultural process, therefore, stigma carries an essentially moral significance that threatens the integrity of the stigmatized individual [6].

In a psychosocial perspective, Goffman's mark or sign is not in itself indicative, but acquires negative significances that are then transferred to the bearer in the course of social interactions [31]. Stigmatization arises when an individual possesses or is likely to possess certain attributes associated with a social identity perceived as devalued in a specific social context [32–36]. Goffman considered that stigma materializes through practice as a powerful social label that represents a severe critique of an individual's attributes in specific social interactions. The construction of stigma as a process dependent on the perception that there exists a normal or standard social identity that does not include those perceived as different or deviant, those who become stigmatized [13]. Researchers proposed that stigma "is the characteristic of a person who does not conform to a social unit in which the norm is defined as a common belief that a person must act a certain way in a given moment [37]." To summarize, these definitions have at their core the shared idea that stigmatized individuals have or may have certain socially devalued attributes [38]. Such stigmatization has been studied in various contexts, including syphilis in the nineteenth century [39], cancer [40], epilepsy [41], poverty and social housing [42], and HIV/AIDS [30, 43–45]. To borrow from Goffman's perspective, therefore, the seemingly indelible mark borne by PLHIV/AIDS translates into an identity distorted by the pandemic.

3. Research into the nature and manifestations of stigma

Kelly et al. produced pioneering research into the relationship between health-care providers and PLHIV/AIDS, suggesting that physicians reacted with negative emotions toward AIDS diagnoses based on presumptions about patients' homosexual promiscuity rather than their sexual orientation as such [46]. Subsequently, a number of studies provided clear evidence of stigmatization within the health-care field in the early years of the history of HIV/AIDS and a fear of providing health care to PLHIV/AIDS [47, 48]. Authors also documented cases of refusal to provide care to PLHIV/AIDS [8] as well as instances of caregivers breaching patient confidentiality [49].

That the first known cases of infection were those of homosexual men tended to lend the disease a sensationalist aspect, not only in the public eye but also within the health-care field more specifically [7]. Homophobic attitudes among physicians thus acquired greater significance [46, 50, 51]. At the beginning of the pandemic, in fact, American physicians perceived HIV/AIDS as more closely related to homosexuality than to other diseases [52]. Research carried out through the early 1990s reveals highly negative attitudes on the part of doctors toward PLHIV/AIDS [8]. Throughout the 1980s and 1990s, a large proportion of health-care personnel remained unaware of the tremendous potency of stigma associated with HIV/AIDS. It was indeed during those two decades that prejudices and negative behaviors were most prevalent among health-care professionals in all affected regions. To be sure, there exists a clear consensus in the literature as to the difficulties PLHIV/AIDS have had to tackle in their relationship with health care during that period. In addition, the conservative public health policies in effect at the time reinforced negative social constructions and set in place marginalized social categories [53]. Clearly, therefore, the two decades that saw the outburst and multiplication of HIV/AIDS cases were characterized by a highly potent stigmatization of PLHIV/AIDS and prevalent fears among health-care personnel, both of which affected the delivery of care to PLHIV/AIDS. Experiences of discrimination and stigmatization in the provision of health care are documented in numerous studies undertaken at the time [9, 49, 54]. By contrast, only a small proportion of studies carried out during the 1990s noted an absence of discrimination toward PLHIV/AIDS on the part of caregivers [55, 56].

Furthermore, the literature provides evidence that behaviors stigmatizing HIV/AIDS observed during the second half of the 1980s continued to be present not only through the 1990s but into the 2000s, as well. Although negative behaviors toward certain marginalized groups in the delivery of HIV/AIDS health care were observed during the 1980s and 1990s [10, 57, 58], researchers all remarked on the presence of negative attitudes on the part of caregivers in relation to such factors as socioeconomic status, mental health, and race. Similar results were

http://dx.doi.org/10.5772/66654

also suggested in another study [57]. In the same vein, other researchers such as Parker [44] have described stigma and discrimination linked to HIV/AIDS as complex social processes that act on one another and reinforce preexisting stigma and discrimination toward sexuality, gender, race, and poverty. For their part [9], in their study of public hospitals in Belize, they found that stigmatizing attitudes and discrimination toward PLHIV/AIDS among health personnel correlated with religious and conservative outlooks, corroborating results reported by other researchers [59, 60] (1989). The most conspicuous components of stigma directed at PLHIV/AIDS were reproach and judgment; moreover, they found that in providing care to PLHIV/AIDS, physicians exhibited more stigmatizing attitudes than did nurses [9]. The authors suggest, furthermore, that the most discernible stigmatizing attitude among doctors was a perception of PLHIV/AIDS as entirely responsible for their own condition. Similarly, the study results [61] indicate that doctors exhibit more pronounced attitudes of refusal toward PLHIV/AIDS than do nurses and hospital support staff.

In a study concerned with Southeast China, they observed that caregivers were less inclined to provide health care to PLHIV/AIDS, corroborating both contemporary studies and others dating to the early 1990s [62]. Within the Chinese health-care system, in addition, regional disparities in HIV/AIDS education, as well as in material resources, appear especially acute and point to deep-rooted problems: the study found that the personnel of village health stations were particularly disinclined to provide services to PLHIV/AIDS. Overall, a significant number of studies covering the period 2000–2012 indicate that stigma directed toward PLHIV/AIDS persists within the health-care field [49, 53, 63–67] and continues to influence the relationship between health personnel and PLHIV/AIDS [11, 23, 68–71]. Ultimately, such attitudes contribute to keep PLHIV/AIDS anonymous and faceless in the eyes of broader society [48].

4. Archetypes as the source of HIV/AIDS stigma

Although the male homosexual population was the first to be targeted as responsible for the disease during the 1980s, researchers observed the presence of a persistent discourse, within the American public health context, attributing a measure of responsibility for the disease's transmission to prostitutes [50]. Such a discourse reproduces and perpetuates representations of deviance that, moreover, are closely linked with perceptions of women as "polluting." Another major theme implicit in significations attached to AIDS that emerges in reference to prostitutes and HIV-positive mothers is that of the self-control and self-discipline of one's body. These representations of the disease, therefore, carry the notion that HIV/AIDS can be avoided through "disciplined" behavior and that, by consequence, those who carry the virus are solely responsible for their infection. The discourse assumes that since there exist ways of avoiding infection, those who become infected are responsible (i.e., guilty) and, as such, undeserving of sympathy (Sacks, 1996). Infection is thus equated with undesirable behaviors, particularly as regards sexual practices. We cannot demonstrate that beliefs determine actions, because both beliefs and actions are expressions of fundamental representations [72]. Researchers [73], for her part, provided a clear illustration of this assertion in her observations of exclusion rituals in homes where a family member suffered from mental illness, including the segregation of their clothing and linens from the rest of the family's laundry. Villagers had adopted these rituals as a way of accepting the mentally ill within the family home without risk of "infecting" their families; local representations held that madness was an infection born of false beliefs.

An analysis of three dominant archetypes at the root of negative significations attached to HIV/AIDS reveals the ways in which discourses, significations, and representations have changed over time [74]. The archetype of the victim of AIDS victim, which first emerged during the 1980s, continued to carry negative significations in the lives of the infected in the mid-1990s. The representations linked with this archetype held that PLHIV/AIDS were ravaged, disfigured, and debilitated by the syndrome, as well as alone, desperate, and condemned to inevitable death [75]. This pessimistic AIDS archetype was increasingly contested during the early 1990s by accounts that presented a divergent, more optimistic vision, culminating in the emergence of the archetype of the AIDS survivor. In contrast to the victim archetype, representations of AIDS survivors were linked with notions of fighting against disease and despair and found their most prominent public incarnation in Earvin "Magic" **Johnson**, the basketball star whose public announcement of his HIV-positive status and subsequent AIDS activism made him a rallying figure (Lupton, 1999). The third dominant archetype in the media in the early 1990s was that of the HIV carrier. The public availability of antiretroviral drugs by 1994 made it possible for people infected with the virus to stave off the development of the syndrome. The representations associated with this change centered on encouraging carriers to live their lives fully while keeping the virus under control through medicine.

In contrast with the archetype of the survivor, the figure of the homosexual was not frequently portrayed as representative of the HIV carrier. The media did, however, associate the HIV carrier archetype with women portrayed as morally suspect, in particular prostitutes and women from disadvantaged backgrounds [50, 76]. This alarmist perception of HIV/AIDS may be understood in terms of epidemic psychology, in which suspicion, fear, and panic emerge as reactions to possible infection when an epidemic is perceived as particularly dangerous to a society [59]. By the mid-1990s, media representations of HIV-positive women engaged in the struggle against AIDS began to show them as integral individuals unencumbered by guilt over their infection with whom the public could identify, rather than as those to be avoided, abused, or judged; in other words, as people living with AIDS, rather than dying from it [76]. This demonstrates the positive representation of women as having power over their situation and expresses the empowerment of HIV-positive women.

The three archetypal representations are linked with stigma, however. The victim of AIDS is represented as a victim also of discrimination and despair. The AIDS survivor is presented in a hopeful light. With the exceptions noted above, the AIDS carrier, by contrast, is represented in a negative light, as having a body that is a source of risk and having permeable boundaries through which the HIV virus can be transmitted to others. It is worth noting that the emergence of the negative archetype of the HIV carrier coincided with the development of the first antiretroviral drugs, which gave rise to a new, positive dimension in the lives of the infected, but, having extended their life, gave rise also to fears of a greater risk that they might pass the virus on to others.

5. The consequences of stigmatizing behavior in health care

A number of studies suggest that refusals to offer care based on prejudices can erect communication barriers and cause confidence to deteriorate, imposing additional limitations on HIV/AIDS medical care [22, 48, 69, 77]. Indeed, stigma is broadly recognized as an important barrier for prevention and treatment of HIV/AIDS [27, 66, 78–81] and as affecting the stigmatized individual's social situation and psychological health [82, 83]. Studies carried out in Thailand have noted that stigmatization of PLHIV/AIDS in the context of medical care constitutes a significant barrier to the delivery of services to PLHIV/AIDS [28]. Similarly, the work reveals points to intentional delays of medical appointments for PLHIV/AIDS, particularly for surgeries, as well as oral and dental care. The study notes that 43% of medical personnel would not consult a dentist who had tested HIV-positive, while 36% indicated a belief that an HIV-positive physician should not be allowed to perform surgeries and a full 65% of administrative personnel insisted on such a ban [64]. Thus, perceptions of PLHIV/AIDS influence their access to appropriate care. Other authors have in addition noted behaviors among medical personnel denoting stigma when interacting with PLHIV/AIDS, including refusal of care, reduced quality of care, as well as ignoring and intimidating patients, exhibiting anger and employing excessive precautions against infection [54, 68], other observed attitudes include pity and disillusion [69], as well as minimal eye contact, distance in conversation, devaluing attitudes, and excessive security measures [12, 68].

However, results reported [48] in a study of PLHIV/AIDS health care in the Maule region of Chile show that more recently health professionals, and physicians in particular, have pointed to a decrease in stigma toward PLHIV/AIDS in health center contexts and that there has been a positive change in the attitudes of physicians toward HIV/AIDS patients. In addition, the study shows that the majority of patient testimonies on the attitudes of caregivers indicate the latter's growing engagement and attention to a whole-person approach to care. These results point to positive changes over time in health-care provision to PLHIV/AIDS. The authors note, as well, that caregiver testimonies indicate that a similar positive change in attitudes toward patients has also permeated other areas of health care. Similarly, a study [84] involving eight HIV/AIDS-positive women of African origin in the city of Nottingham, England, shows that participants described health services as a safe social space and a source of positive support. Other results, however, suggest that when caregivers report experiencing positive emotions toward patients, it is overwhelmingly toward those who represent populations traditionally considered to be the pandemic's "innocent" victims, such as children or women infected by their partners [69] underlining a development over time in stigma directed toward those perceived as innocent [63] or faultless [80] in contrast to those seen as "guilty" patients [20, 50, 76, 85].

Our overview of the relatively short history of HIV/AIDS and the research literature concerned with various aspects of the pandemic underscores the scope and persistence of stigmatization across a range of practices. The stigmatizing attitudes described above are founded in specific discourses and representations, and can range from an indifferent gesture to a convinced decision, from passive negligence to violent rejection. We have also observed, however, that positive attitudes appear to be progressing in certain HIV/AIDS health-care environments. The distance between caregivers and patients has lessened over time, as evidenced by patient testimonies of positive experiences in interactions with health services. The result is that the health-care space, which was once a source of concern for PLHIV/AIDS, has begun to acquire a more positive significance through more inclusive care practices and behaviors that better serve those in need. What is more, the concept of offering PLHIV/AIDS a care relationship that goes beyond strictly medical needs has also begun to take root among clinicians. Health workers increasingly view the disease as requiring a whole-person approach that is apt to more fully address a range of social and moral impacts in the lives of PLHIV/AIDS [48].

6. Conclusion

This review of the literature on the stigmatization of PLHIV/AIDS, in a variety of health-care contexts since the outbreak of the pandemic in the 1980s, provides evidence for the persistence of social stigma toward the infected, but also shows that stigma is attenuated or reduced in certain social settings and where specifically dedicated care is accessible [48, 84]. In the reviewed literature, the notion of stigmatization covers a wide range of psychosocial phenomena (attitudes and behaviors of caregivers) and perceptions (those of both caregivers and patients) that require a more comprehensive conceptual definition of stigma and the process of stigmatization than has been offered to date. The perspective developed by Goffman, which focuses on interaction frameworks, provides solid footing on which to develop an understanding of the nature and manifestations of stigmatization in the specific context of health services. Inquiries into the interactions between medical personnel and PLHIV/AIDS are likely to be particularly fruitful. At present, studies taking into account the perceptions of both PLHIV/AIDS and caregivers are exceedingly rare [86]. While existing studies rely primarily on analyses of respondents' testimonies of experiences, in vivo observations of interactions appear more apt to produce comprehensive results for understanding stigmatization processes.

In terms of the effects of stigmatizing behaviors on the provision of care to PLHIV/AIDS, although some studies show an improvement in attitudes on the part of caregivers PLHIV/AIDS [48, 84], the majority of the literature does not suggest a unilateral shift from a period of stigmatization to one of widespread compassion and social solidarity with the infected [4–6, 9–11]. The reduction of stigma toward HIV/AIDS and its consequences was identified as an important goal by the UN as far back as the year 2000 (Elliott, 2002). Yet, existing health policies still do not, or only inadequately, address PLHIV/AIDS stigmatization by health personnel. Many health policies remain framed in a population health perspective that only occasionally acknowledges the prejudices, stereotypes, and discrimination that PLHIV/AIDS may face in society.

Furthermore, the literature reviewed above is concerned largely with medical personnel in the context of modern health-care organizational structures in which work is divided along hierarchical lines of professional classification. Within this diversity of professions and areas of care, preventive and therapeutic interventions related to HIV/AIDS have varied consider-

http://dx.doi.org/10.5772/66654

ably since the first positive diagnoses and subsequent development of monotherapy treatments in the early 1980s. In order to better understand stigmatization, it is necessary to link the perceptions of health professionals on PLHIV/AIDS with broader social beliefs about disease, on both the social and individual levels, in relation to public policies and clinical interventions. While a majority of studies appear to consider categories of caregivers as mutually independent units, in practice interventions happen within multipurpose institutions staffed by multidisciplinary teams of caregivers. Preventive and therapeutic outlooks are elaborated within teams that span different professional categories, based on a number of shared postulates, in the course of discussions on specific courses of action in specific cases. It seems important therefore to further examine changes in the stigma and related behaviors associated with HIV/AIDS in specific professional contexts rather than in specific professional categories.

Thanks to biomedical research, HIV/AIDS has today become a chronic, rather than fatal, disease. Yet, indicators of the persistence of stigma directed at HIV/AIDS in health-care contexts suggest that the various components of caregiver-PLHIV/AIDS interactions are yet to be fully understood. Studies conducted in a range of social and cultural contexts demonstrate the persistence of negative (and potentially stigmatizing) behaviors toward PLHIV/AIDS in the field of health care. The results of the present examination of continuing stigma represent, therefore, a valuable contribution to the literature and point the way to further research.

Author details

Oscar Labra* and Daniel Thomas

*Address all correspondence to: oscar.labra@uqat.ca

Department of Human and Social Development, Université du Québec en Abitibi-Témiscamingue, Canada

References

[1] Desclaux, A., Stigmatisation, discrimination: que peut-on attendre d'une approche culturelle? 2003.

[2] Bettega, N., Social representation of AIDS among Zambian adolescents. Journal of Health Psychology, 2003. 8(5): pp. 616–631.

[3] Brasileiro, M. and Freitas, M.I.d.F., Social representations about aids in people over 50, infected by HIV. Revista Latino-americana de Enfermagem, 2006. 14(5): pp. 789–795.

[4] Chao, L.W., et al., HIV/AIDS stigma attitudes among educators in KwaZulu-Natal, South Africa. Journal of School Health, 2010. 80(11): pp. 561–569.

[5] Brown, D.C., BeLue, R., and Airhihenbuwa, C.O., HIV and AIDS-related stigma in the context of family support and race in South Africa. Ethnicity & Health, 2010. 15(5): pp. 441–458.

[6] Yang, L.H., et al., Culture and stigma: adding moral experience to stigma theory. Social Science & Medicine, 2007. 64(7): pp. 1524–1535.

[7] Moatti, J., et al., Social perception of AIDS in the general public: a French study. Health Policy, 1988. 9(1): pp. 1–8.

[8] Gerbert, B., et al., Physicians and AIDS. Journal of General Internal Medicine, 1992. 7(6): pp. 657–664.

[9] Andrewin, A. and Chien, L.-Y., Stigmatization of patients with HIV/AIDS among doctors and nurses in Belize. AIDS Patient Care and STDs, 2008. 22(11): pp. 897–906.

[10] Logie, C., et al., Associations between HIV-related stigma, racial discrimination, gender discrimination, and depression among HIV-positive African, Caribbean, and Black women in Ontario, Canada. AIDS Patient Care and STDs, 2013. 27(2): pp. 114–122.

[11] Olowookere, S. and Adewole, I., Socio-demographic characteristics and challenges experienced by disabled patients living with HIV/AIDS in a tertiary hospital in Ibadan, Nigeria. African Journal of Medicine and Medical Sciences, 2012. 41(3): pp. 243–248.

[12] Labra, O., Social representations of HIV/AIDS in mass media: some important lessons for caregivers. International Social Work, 2015. 58(2): pp. 238–248.

[13] Erving Goffman, S., Notes on the Management of Spoiled Identity. Englewood Cliffs, NJ: Prentice-Hall, 1963.

[14] Saillant, F., Cancer et Culture. Montréal: Les Éditions Saint-Martin, 1988.

[15] Castro, A. and Farmer, P., Violence structurelle, mondialisation et tuberculose multi-résistante. Anthropologie et Sociétés, 2003. 27(2): pp. 23–40.

[16] Gilman, S.L., AIDS and syphilis: the iconography of disease. 1987. 43: pp. 87–107.

[17] Markova, I. and Wilkie, P., Representations, concepts and social change: the phenomenon of AIDS. Journal for the Theory of Social Behaviour, 1987. 17(4): pp. 389–409.

[18] Taerk, G., et al., Recurrent themes of concern in groups for health care professionals. AIDS Care, 1993. 5(2): pp. 215–222.

[19] McCann, T.V. and Sharkey, R.J., Educational intervention with international nurses and changes in knowledge, attitudes and willingness to provide care to patients with HIV/AIDS. Journal of Advanced Nursing, 1998. 27(2): pp. 267–273.

[20] Herek, G.M., et al., Workshop report: AIDS and stigma: a conceptual framework and research agenda. AIDS & Public Policy Journal, 1998. 13(1): p. 36.

http://dx.doi.org/10.5772/66654

[21] Uwakwe, C.B., Systematized HIV/AIDS education for student nurses at the University of Ibadan, Nigeria: impact on knowledge, attitudes and compliance with universal precautions. Journal of Advanced Nursing, 2000. 32(2): pp. 416–424.

[22] Bray Preston, D., et al., Personal and social determinants of rural nurses' willingness to care for persons with AIDS. Research in Nursing & Health, 2000. 23(1): pp. 67–78.

[23] Taylor, B., HIV, stigma and health: integration of theoretical concepts and the lived experiences of individuals. Journal of Advanced Nursing, 2001. 35(5): pp. 792–798.

[24] Zelaya, C.E., et al., HIV/AIDS stigma: reliability and validity of a new measurement instrument in Chennai, India. AIDS and Behavior, 2008. 12(5): pp. 781–788.

[25] Elford, J., et al., HIV-related discrimination reported by people living with HIV in London, UK. AIDS and Behavior, 2008. 12(2): pp. 255–264.

[26] Riley, G.A. and Baah-Odoom, D., Do stigma, blame and stereotyping contribute to unsafe sexual behaviour? A test of claims about the spread of HIV/AIDS arising from social representation theory and the AIDS risk reduction model. Social Science & Medicine, 2010. 71(3): pp. 600–607.

[27] Chan, K.Y. and Reidpath, D.D., Stigmatization of patients with AIDS: understanding the interrelationships between Thai nurses' attitudes toward HIV/AIDS, drug use, and commercial sex. AIDS Patient Care and STDs, 2007. 21(10): pp. 763–775.

[28] Chan, K.Y., et al., Stigmatization of AIDS patients: disentangling Thai nursing students' attitudes towards HIV/AIDS, drug use, and commercial sex. AIDS and Behavior, 2008. 12(1): pp. 146–157.

[29] Teixeira, M.G. and Silva, G.A.d., Representation of the HIV carriers about antiretroviral treatment. Revista da Escola de Enfermagem da USP, 2008. 42(4): pp. 729–736.

[30] Stephenson, P.H., Le sida, la syphilis et la stigmatisation. La genèse des politiques et des préjugés. Anthropologie et Sociétés, 1991. 15(2–3): pp. 91–104.

[31] Herek, G.M., Beyond "homophobia": thinking about sexual prejudice and stigma in the twenty-first century. Sexuality Research & Social Policy, 2004. 1(2): pp. 6–24.

[32] Sellers, R.M. and Shelton, J.N., The role of racial identity in perceived racial discrimination. Journal of Personality and Social Psychology, 2003. 84(5): p. 1079.

[33] Taylor, J. and Turner, R.J., Perceived discrimination, social stress, and depression in the transition to adulthood: racial contrasts. Social Psychology Quarterly, 2002: pp. 213–225.

[34] Steele, C.M., A threat in the air: how stereotypes shape intellectual identity and performance. American Psychologist, 1997. 52(6): p. 613.

[35] Crocker, J., Cornwell, B., and Major, B., The stigma of overweight: affective consequences of attributional ambiguity. Journal of Personality and Social Psychology, 1993. 64(1): p. 60.

[36] Jones, E.E., Social Stigma: The Psychology of Marked Relationships. WH Freeman, 1984.

[37] Stafford, M.C. and Scott, R.R., Stigma, deviance, and social control, in The Dilemma of Difference. Springer, 1986, pp. 77–91.

[38] Major, B. and O'Brien, L.T., The social psychology of stigma. Annual Review of Psychology, 2005. 56: pp. 393–421.

[39] Claude, Q., Le mal de Naples. Histoire de la syphilis. Paris: Seghers, 1986.

[40] Fife, B.L. and Wright, E.R., The dimensionality of stigma: a comparison of its impact on the self of persons with HIV/AIDS and cancer. Journal of Health and Social Behavior, 2000: pp. 50–67.

[41] Schneider, J.W. and Conrad, P., In the closet with illness: epilepsy, stigma potential and information control. Social Problems, 1980. 28(1): pp. 32–44.

[42] Dansereau, F., Villemaire, L., and Archambault, J., Le logement social et la lutte contre la pauvreté et l'exclusion sociale. 2002: Institut national de la recherche scientifique, Urbanisation, Culture et Société.

[43] Fay, C., Risques, enjeux et partenaires de la lutte internationale contre le sida. Autrepart, 1999. 12: pp. 5–17.

[44] Parker, R. and Aggleton, P., HIV and AIDS-related stigma and discrimination: a conceptual framework and implications for action. Social Science & Medicine, 2003. 57(1): pp. 13–24.

[45] d'Île-de-France, O.r.d.l.s., Sida, A.n.d.r.s.l., and Halfen, S., Les connaissances, attitudes, croyances et comportements face au VIH/sida aux Antilles et en Guyane en 2004. Observatoire régional de la santé d'Île-de-France, 2006.

[46] Kelly, J.A., et al., Stigmatization of AIDS patients by physicians. American Journal of Public Health, 1987. 77(7): pp. 789–791.

[47] Knox, M. and Dow, M., Staff discomfort in working with HIV spectrum patients. in 5th International Conference on AIDS, Montreal, Canada. 1989.

[48] Labra, Ó. and Dumont, S., Representaciones sociales del VIH-SIDA en la Región del Maule, Chile. Revista de Trabajo Social, 2012. (83): pp. 35–40.

[49] Surlis, S. and Hyde, A., HIV-positive patients' experiences of stigma during hospitalization. Journal of the Association of Nurses in AIDS Care, 2001. 12(6): pp. 68–77.

[50] Sacks, V., Women and AIDS: an analysis of media misrepresentations. Social Science & Medicine, 1996. 42(1): pp. 59–73.

[51] Norton, R., Schwartzbaum, J., and Wheat, J., Language discrimination of general physicians FIS metaphors used in the AIDS crisis. Communication Research, 1990. 17(6): pp. 809–826.

[52] Joffe, H., AIDS research and prevention: a social representational approach. British Journal of Medical Psychology, 1996. 69(3): pp. 169–190.

[53] Rutledge, S.E., et al., AIDS stigma in health services in the Eastern Caribbean. Sociology of Health & Illness, 2009. 31(1): pp. 17–34.

[54] Rahmati-Najarkolaei, F., et al., Experiences of stigma in healthcare settings among adults living with HIV in the Islamic Republic of Iran. Journal of the International AIDS Society, 2010. 13(1): p. 27.

[55] Katz, M.H., et al., Insurance type and satisfaction with medical care among HIV-infected men. JAIDS Journal of Acquired Immune Deficiency Syndromes, 1997. 14(1): pp. 35–43.

[56] Green, G. and Platt, S., Fear and loathing in health care settings reported by people with HIV. Sociology of Health & Illness, 1997. 19(1): pp. 70–92.

[57] Bird, S.T., Bogart, L.M., and Delahanty, D.L., Health-related correlates of perceived discrimination in HIV care. AIDS Patient Care and STDs, 2004. 18(1): pp. 19–26.

[58] Logie, C. and Gadalla, T., Meta-analysis of health and demographic correlates of stigma towards people living with HIV. AIDS Care, 2009. 21(6): pp. 742–753.

[59] Strong, P., Epidemic psychology: a model. Sociology of Health & Illness, 1990. 12(3): pp. 249–259.

[60] Echabe, A.E. and Rovira, D.P., Social representations and memory: the case of AIDS. European Journal of Social Psychology, 1989. 19(6): pp. 543–551.

[61] Mahendra, V.S., et al., Understanding and measuring AIDS-related stigma in health care settings: a developing country perspective. SAHARA-J: Journal of Social Aspects of HIV/AIDS, 2007. 4(2): pp. 616–625.

[62] Cai, G., et al., Inequality and unwillingness to care for people living with HIV/AIDS: a survey of medical professionals in Southeast China. AIDS Patient Care and STDs, 2007. 21(8): pp. 593–601.

[63] Zukoski, A.P. and Thorburn, S., Experiences of stigma and discrimination among adults living with HIV in a low HIV-prevalence context: a qualitative analysis. AIDS Patient Care and STDs, 2009. 23(4): pp. 267–276.

[64] Infante, C., et al., HIV/AIDS-related stigma and discrimination: the case of health care providers in Mexico. Salud Publica de Mexico, 2006. 48(2): pp. 141–150.

[65] Sullivan, L.M., et al., The doctor–patient relationship and HIV-infected patients' satisfaction with primary care physicians. Journal of General Internal Medicine, 2000. 15(7): pp. 462–469.

[66] Fiscella, K., et al., Patient trust: is it related to patient-centered behavior of primary care physicians? Medical Care, 2004. 42(11): pp. 1049–1055.

[67] Li, L., et al., Stigmatization and shame: consequences of caring for HIV/AIDS patients in China. AIDS Care, 2007. 19(2): pp. 258–263.

[68] Rintamaki, L.S., et al., Male patient perceptions of HIV stigma in health care contexts. AIDS Patient Care and STDs, 2007. 21(12): pp. 956–969.

[69] Varas-Diaz, N. and Marzan-Rodriguez, M., The emotional aspect of AIDS stigma among health professionals in Puerto Rico. AIDS Care, 2007. 19(10): pp. 1247–1257.

[70] Lekas, H.-M., Siegel, K., and Schrimshaw, E.W., Continuities and discontinuities in the experiences of felt and enacted stigma among women with HIV/AIDS. Qualitative Health Research, 2006. 16(9): pp. 1165–1190.

[71] Li, L., et al., Reducing HIV-related stigma in health care settings: a randomized controlled trial in China. American Journal of Public Health, 2013. 103(2): pp. 286–292.

[72] Wagner, W., The fallacy of misplaced intentionality in social representation research. Journal for the Theory of Social Behaviour, 1994. 24(3): pp. 243–165.

[73] Jodelet, D., Les Représentations Sociales. Presses universitaires de France, 2003.

[74] Chapman, E., Patient impact of negative representations of HIV. AIDS Patient Care and STDs, 2002. 16(4): pp. 173–177.

[75] Lupton, D., Archetypes of infection: people with HIV/AIDS in the Australian press in the mid 1990s. Sociology of Health & Illness, 1999. 21(1): pp. 37–53.

[76] Juhasz, A., The contained threat: women in mainstream AIDS documentary. Journal of Sex Research, 1990. 27(1): pp. 25–46.

[77] Curtis, J.R., et al., Why don't patients and physicians talk about end-of-life care? Barriers to communication for patients with acquired immunodeficiency syndrome and their primary care clinicians. Archives of Internal Medicine, 2000. 160(11): pp. 1690–1696.

[78] Airhihenbuwa, C., Healing Our Differences: The Global Crisis of Health and Politics of Identity. 2007, Rowman and Littlefield, Lanham, MD.

[79] Simbayi, L.C., et al., Internalized stigma, discrimination, and depression among men and women living with HIV/AIDS in Cape Town, South Africa. Social Science & Medicine, 2007. 64(9): pp. 1823–1831.

[80] McCann, T.V., Willingness to provide care and treatment for patients with HIV/AIDS. Journal of Advanced Nursing, 1997. 25(5): pp. 1033–1039.

[81] Kinsler, J.J., et al., The effect of perceived stigma from a health care provider on access to care among a low-income HIV-positive population. AIDS Patient Care and STDs, 2007. 21(8): pp. 584–592.

[82] Crandall, C.S. and Eshleman, A., A justification-suppression model of the expression and experience of prejudice. Psychological Bulletin, 2003. 129(3): p. 414.

http://dx.doi.org/10.5772/66654

[83] Crandall, C.S., Do parents discriminate against their heavyweight daughters? Personality and Social Psychology Bulletin, 1995. 21: pp. 724–724.

[84] Ndirangu, E.W. and Evans, C., Experiences of African immigrant women living with HIV in the UK: implications for health professionals. Journal of Immigrant and Minority Health, 2009. 11(2): pp. 108–114.

[85] Herek, G.M., Widaman, K.F., and Capitanio, J.P., When sex equals AIDS: symbolic stigma and heterosexual adults' inaccurate beliefs about sexual transmission of AIDS. Social Problems, 2005. 52(1): pp. 15–37.

[86] Wallach, I., et al., Le VIH et le vieillissement au Québec. Une recherche qualitative sur les expériences, les difficultés et les besoins des personnes vivant avec le VIH de 50 ans et plus. Nous, 2012.

Chapter 8

Economic Globalization, HIV and AIDS and Gender Dimensions in the Lesotho Textiles and Garment Industry

Pius Tangwe Tanga, Haruna M. Bello,
Tiisetso J. Makatjane and Tumelo Tsikoane

Additional information is available at the end of the chapter

http://dx.doi.org/10.5772/66653

Abstract

The Kingdom of Lesotho is also experiencing the third highest HIV and AIDS prevalence rate (23.2%) in the world, which poses an internal threat both to the industry and to the workers. The objective of this chapter was to examine workers' economic opportunities, the interplay of HIV and AIDS as well as threats to economic opportunities provided by the industry. This chapter is based on data collected for a study on the economic crisis, globalization and HIV and AIDS nexus in the textiles and garment industry in Lesotho. Data for this chapter were generated from two of the three instruments of the main study using a multistage sampling technique. Data collected were analysed quantitatively using Statistical Package for the Social Sciences (SPSS). The result shows that despite the economic crisis, the textiles and garment industry has enhanced the employment of many *Basotho* (people from Lesotho), especially women. Although workers were economically empowered, HIV and AIDS and the global economic crisis were threats to the industry and workers alike. There is significant rural-urban migration to the industry with almost half of the workers staying away from their traditional family homes.

Keywords: economic globalisation, HIV and AIDS, textiles and garment industry, Lesotho, global economic crisis

1. Introduction

Lesotho is predominantly a mountainous country, with an altitude range of between 1300 and 3500 masl (over 80% of the land is over 1800 m altitude) [1]. The surface area of Lesotho is approximately 30,350 km^2 demarcated into 10 administrative districts. One-quarter of the land is lowlands and the remainder is highlands. Only 9% of the total area is suitable for arable cultivation. Lesotho is described as one of the poorest countries in Sub-Saharan Africa (SSA) with an estimated population of 1.8 million [2]. The majority of the population (77%) resides in the rural and mountainous areas [3, 4]. Lesotho has four seasons with the mountainous areas experiencing heavy snowfall during winters sometimes resulting in loss of livestock and making accessibility to the urban areas almost impossible.

The country has few natural resource endowments but has abundance of labour, water and beautiful landscape whose economic potential remains untapped. There are also concentrations of diamonds. The country enjoys royalties from export of water to the Republic of South Africa (RSA) and remittances resulting from labour migration constituted 28% of the country's GDP in 2010. However, the mine workers have been experiencing increasing retrenchment from the South African mines resulting in an unemployment figure estimated at 45% [5]. This notwithstanding, labour migration, government and textiles and garment industry are the three main forms of employment in the country [3].

The country is faced with a number of challenges but unemployment, HIV and AIDS and retrenchments of Basotho men by the South African mining industry are the main ones. Retrenchments from South African mining industry and the decline in engaging young Basotho men as labour migrants contributed to the high unemployment rate of 45% in 2010 in the country. Employment created by textiles and garment industry is likely to surpass employment created by government in the future hence the need to investigate the impact of economic globalisation on the textiles and garment industry. Furthermore, since the textile and garment industry is a major employer of women (over 70%) in the economy, it is imperative to investigate the nexus between HIV/AIDS and employment in the textile and garment industry in the face of the then on-going economic globalization trend.

Lesotho does not only have the third highest prevalence of HIV and AIDS in the world after Botswana and Swaziland [3, 6–8]; it has also prioritised reduction of HIV as its number one priority among the Millennium Development Goals (MDGs). Available statistics indicate that HIV prevalence sharply increased from around 4% in 1993, to 25% in 1999 and to an estimated 31% in 2002 [9]. According to the 2004 and 2009 Lesotho Demographic Household Survey (DHS) figures, HIV prevalence in Lesotho has remained high at around 23% [10]. It is not surprising that in 2000, HIV was declared a crisis in Lesotho. According to the Ministry of Health and Social Welfare (MoHSW) [11] in the Demographic Health Survey of 2009, it was found that concurrent and multiple sexual partnership is a common feature in Lesotho's society [10]. Six percent of women and 21% of men have had more than two sexual partners in the last 12 months. Within these figures, condom use was only 39% of females and 52% of men having reported using a condom during their last sexual encounter, suggesting unequal sexual power relations disadvantages women in the spread of HIV/AIDS through sexual intercourse [10, 11].

Among a number of attempts to curb the spread of HIV the Lesotho AIDS Programme Coordinating Authority (LAPCA) was established within the office of the Prime Minister in

2001 to coordinate national efforts to address the HIV epidemic. In 2005, the National AIDS Commission (NAC) was established to coordinate implementation of the National HIV and AIDS Strategic Plan, thus superseding LAPCA. An in-depth review of the national response in 2005 resulted in an updated National AIDS Policy and the National Strategic Plan for 2006–2011 as well as the approval of the National Monitoring and Evaluation Plan by the Government of Lesotho (GOL) in December 2006 [12]. Lesotho has also shown consistent political leadership on HIV and AIDS. Since the declaration of HIV and AIDS as an emergency in 2000, the top political leadership has consistently spoken out and supported the HIV and AIDS response at the highest level. At the work place, employers are expected to have HIV policies to address HIV and AIDS issues at the work place including the fight against stigmatization and discrimination.

The Senkatana Centre was opened in 2004 to provide antiretroviral therapy (ART) in the country. In 2005, an HIV paediatric clinical centre—the Baylor-Bristol-Myers Squibb Centre of Excellence—was also opened. Baylor provides state-of-the-art facilities for testing, treating and monitoring patients and training healthcare professionals. At the end of 2007, an estimated 21,710 people were receiving anti-retroviral treatment and the coverage of Prevention of Mother-to-Child Transmission (PMTCT) programmes had increased six-fold from an estimated 5% in 2005 to 31% in 2007 [3]. "Know Your Status" (KYS) campaign was also launched in 2004. In 2007, an estimated 12% of the population had received an HIV test in Lesotho representing a threefold increase from the 2005 figures [7].

Access to the US market under the African Growth and Opportunity Act (AGOA) that made Lesotho the single largest beneficiary from Africa has led to increased employment in the textiles and garment industry [13]. The textiles sector employed about 50,000 workers in 2003/2004, but this significantly declined to 26,475 workers in 2006 [9, 14]. These changes are said to be explained by expiration of preferential trade agreements (PTAs) to which Lesotho has been a beneficiary and the global economic/financial crisis that hit the region in 2007/2008. In 2008, unemployment rate was estimated at 22.7%, of which 21.2% were males against 24.6% females compared to 27.3% in 1999. Economic globalisation could be behind the fluctuations in the employment figures of the textiles and garment industry, hence the interest in how economic globalisation and HIV and AIDS are affecting the textiles and garment industry in Lesotho given that majority of the workers (over 70%) are female with unequal safe and protective sexual power relations. In a study to challenge mainstream theories which present globalization and associated forces as gender neutral, Metcalfe and Rees [15] provide a critical combination of the complexity and interconnections between gender, organization and globalization. The chapter identifies that key stakeholders (transnational corporations, international nongovernmental organizations and government state machineries) need to engage in human rights awareness, equality awareness and raising equality consciousness.

However, the argument pertaining to globalization could be understood in different contexts by different contributors. For example, Townsend, Giorgio, Zembe, Cheyip and Mathews [16] argue that the spread of HIV and AIDS pandemic is closely connected to the process of globalization in the South, and in particular, in Africa where the process happens when human bodies move across borders in search of new economic and educational opportunities or in search of lives free from political conflict and violence. These migrants therefore carry the virus that causes AIDS and often they spread the virus at their destinations. On the other hand, Altman [17] and Tanga [8] state that HIV and AIDS are linked to globalization in a number of ways including the fact that a globalized economy means that vagaries of the market also impact upon spread of infection. The impact of HIV and AIDS is linked to social and economic upheavals which have effectively increased the vulnerability of women, who are more likely to be unable to protect themselves against infection and to carry a greater share of care for those who are sick or infected.

Sapkota [18] conducted a content analysis to identify the degree of mainstreaming of the key elements of globalization in Poverty Reduction Strategy papers in the Asia Pacific region. Trade openness gained the highest priority followed by foreign investment, aid, tourism and lastly migration. Altman [19] and Hirsch [20] highlighted that globalisation has an impact on all aspects of life including sexuality. Sexuality is affected by globalisation in a number of interconnected ways and therefore increases inequalities, acting both as a liberator and an oppressive influence. Pearson [21] argues that people working on gender development in the last third quarter of the twentieth century will lead to the new century realizing the global relevance of gender in development and see that gender analysis is applied in new contexts and to both men and women. According to Sen [22], as quoted by Pearson [21], indications are that the new century will witness an assertion of the global relevance of gender in development institutions and organizations concerned with meeting the challenges of globalisation.

Table 1 shows some socio-economic indicators of Lesotho. With a population of 1.8 million inhabitants, Lesotho has an urbanized population of 25%. Life expectancy has dropped from more than 50 years in the 1990s to 44.9 years in 2008. Furthermore, population poverty line also deteriorated to 56.7%, with a Human Development Index (HDI) ranking of 156 of 182 countries, a GDP per capita of M4795 and an inflation rate of 4.2%. Other important indicators include unemployment figure of 45% as well as high number of orphaned children. The combinations of high levels of poverty and unemployment coupled with high HIV and AIDS prevalence in a population with female majority and an industry that is dependent on female workforce certainly leaves a lot to be desired in terms of the vulnerability that women will go through as a result of global economic crisis.

The objective of this chapter was therefore to review the gender dimensions and interconnectedness of globalization, economic crisis and HIV/AIDS in the textile and garment industry in the Kingdom of Lesotho following the economic financial meltdown of 2008–2009. More specifically, the study aimed to investigate and determine the role of the textile and garment industry as provider of employment opportunities and the nexus between globalization, economic meltdown and HIV/AIDS crisis; determine if HIV/AIDS is an economic threat to the textile and garment industry; and determine if there is a differential in HIV/AIDS vulnerability in the industry based on gender.

http://dx.doi.org/10.5772/66653

Indicator	Value	Year	Source
Population size *(de jure)*	1,862,860	2006	[2]
Population urbanised (%)	23	2006	[2]
Life expectancy at birth	41.2	2006	[14]
Population below poverty line (%)	56.7	2002/3	[23]
Adult (15–49) prevalence of HIV (%)	23.0	2009	[24]
Infant mortality rate (per 1000 live births)	64.6	2007	[25]
Under five mortality rate (per 1000 live births)	98.2	2007	[25]
Maternal mortality rate (per 100,000 live births)	762	2004	[25]
Human Development Index Rank (out of 182 countries)	156	2009	[26]
Population using improved drinking water sources (%)	79	2004	[25]
Population using adequate sanitation facilities (%)	37	2004	[25]
Orphans, children (0–7 years) due to AIDS	130,000	2009	[27]
Orphans, children (0–7 years) due to all causes	200,000	2009	[27]
Crude birth rate per 1000 population	29	2007	[25]
Crude death rate per 1000 population	19.2	2007	[25]
Total fertility rate	3.4	2007	[25]
Skilled attendant at delivery (%)	55.4	1990–2005	[25]
Inflation rate (%)	5.5	2011	[28]
Unemployment rate (%)	45	2010	[5]
GDP growth rate	4.4	2008	[29]
GDP per capita at constant prices (Maloti)	4795	2008	[29]

Table 1. Some socio-economic indicators of Lesotho.

2. Literature review

2.1. Gender dimensions of HIV and AIDS

According to the Ministry of Health and Social Welfare (MoHSW), the bulk of HIV infections in Lesotho have been primarily through heterosexual contact [30] while the National HIV and AIDS Strategic Plan for 2006–2011 reports that the HIV and AIDS epidemic in Lesotho is characterized by high mortality rate estimated at 70 deaths per day, with a resultant increasing number of orphans and vulnerable children [8, 31, 32]. The social, cultural and behavioural factors also contribute to the spread of HIV through concurrent and multiple sexual partnerships [33]. This can better be understood by contextualizing the problem with gender lens. According to Camlin, Kwena, Dworkin, Cohen and Bukusi [34], Sub-Saharan Africa is the only part of the world where HIV prevalence and AIDS deaths are higher for women than for men. They therefore emphasized that gender dimension is crucial to understanding how HIV is spread. The concept facilitates an analysis of how men's and women's roles increase vulnerability to the disease. This is relevant to the Lesotho textiles and garment industry with over 70% of its workforce who are females. Curtis [35] provides a framework for the analysis of the dimension of human diseases within the context of human disease ecology as posited by Meade and Earikson [36]. This context has direct bearing on the gender dimension of HIV and AIDS in Lesotho especially in the textiles and garment industry. They employed the human disease ecology framework to carry out social analysis of HIV and AIDS epidemic in Lesotho highlighting the link between gender inequalities and health. Hlalele and Letsie [37] concluded that there is a general trend in gender inequalities relating to power relations, socialization and cultures as well as legislation in which women remain largely disadvantaged. Nattrass [38] explored the gender dimensions of access to highly active antiretroviral therapy (HAART) in South Africa. Using regression analysis, Natrass found that women are more vulnerable to HIV than men. As a result women access HAART in disproportionately larger numbers compared to men. The findings revealed that fewer men access HAART than women because men in general do not seek treatment for poor health as compared to women. In addition, gender norm makes it difficult for men to admit any health-related weakness and seek medical attention. A number of authors have identified gender inequality as a major driver for the spread of HIV and AIDS [8, 39–42]. Similar views were expressed by Epstein et al. [43] and Mitchell et al. [44] Tanga and Tangwe [9] who claim that gender inequalities fuel HIV and AIDS pandemic and make women more vulnerable to infection. Thus, from the foregoing, understanding the interplay of economic globalization and HIV and AIDS in the textile and garment industry in Lesotho calls for a thorough understanding of the gender dimension in the industry. In the context of Lesotho, socio-cultural differences and power relations between males and females may create gender imbalance in the industry that may predispose women to more vulnerability to the epidemic. Hlalele and Letsie [37] contend that gender inequality and gender-based violence could be promoted by low socio-economic and legal position of women. According to them, this could further be exacerbated by intergenerational sex especially between older males and younger women as a result of their socio-economic vulnerability which appear preponderant in the industry.

Poulsen [45] investigated the gendered impact of HIV and AIDs in South Africa and Swaziland under the auspice of Save the Children. The investigation focused on determining the number and characteristics of children who drop out of school in communities affected by HIV and AIDs as well as primary reasons for drop outs. The result revealed that in most schools teachers acknowledged that HIV and AIDS was a serious issue, particularly in terms of growing numbers of orphans as well as children with sick parents. Parental death was found to be the major cause of disruption of children's home lives. Parental death makes family to be poorer leading children to engage in risky behaviour and more likely to drop out of school. In another study, Bajaj [46] investigated how young women are finding ways to cope with being trapped in a context characterized by severe economic decline and an extensive HIV and AIDS crisis by having "sugar daddies" (rich men). However, the strategies of securing "sugar daddies" result in deadly infection and social isolation of these young women. These studies point to the vulnerability of women and children to the pandemic through unequal power relations. Mindry

http://dx.doi.org/10.5772/66653

[47] thus contends that there is a need to address the HIV crisis in African countries by examining the process in terms of engagement. However, Jewkes [48] recommends that the changes that are needed in school environment should be effective to serve as places for changing sexual practices and gender norms because they are largely the same needed to provide effective education for development. Much more emphasis needs to be given to scaling up delivery interventions to youths in contexts where the curriculum content, skills emphasis, duration, selection of facilitator, use of participatory methods and broader context can be employed.

A baseline study commissioned by the Apparel Lesotho Alliance to Fight AIDS (ALAFA) which assessed the situation of HIV and AIDS among workers in the textile and garment industry in Lesotho revealed a staggering 43.2% rate of prevalence [8, 49]. Further analysis of this study shows that women were significantly more vulnerable than men, with infection levels of 44.2% against 35.6% for men. This finding is important not only due to the significance of the textile and garment industry to the economy of Lesotho but also on account of the demographics of the labour force in the industry where the majority of the workforce are women aged 25–39 years, the age group which has been shown throughout Sub-Saharan Africa to be particularly more vulnerable to HIV infection [4].

2.2. Economic structure, trade and exports

Historic trends of gross domestic product (GDP) growth indicate that Lesotho has performed relatively well over the past two decades, except for 1998 when civil unrest nearly rotted the country [50]. The GDP growth has averaged 3.9% between 1980 and 2006 and stood at 4.4% in 2009. However, challenges still remain. In the past two decades, Lesotho experienced economic transition and has diversified its economy to source growth from other sectors, mainly water development, tourism, manufacturing and mining [51]. Kim et al. [52] identified seven countries in sub-Saharan Africa (Mauritius, Lesotho, South Africa, Madagascar, Kenya, Swaziland and Zimbabwe) as being major exporters of textiles and apparel. They argue that textile and apparel industry is the gate of choice for most countries in the quest to step into industrialization. The US trade policies have been the common factor for the flourishing of the textile and apparel industry in scores of countries of developing countries. It is therefore argued that for the industry to be successful, there should be combined efforts of the local government's industrial and trade policies, the entrepreneurial prowess of the private sector and the flexibility and the work ethic of the labour force. It is on this account that Lesotho took advantage of the African Growth and Opportunity Act (AGOA) to become the largest exporter of garments to the USA from SSA. Exports totalled over $320 million in 2002 [13]. The sector has been an important contributor to economic growth and employment creation. For instance, it contributed about 8% of GDP in the 1980s and reached as high as 16.2% in 2004 [53]. However, despite these positive developments, the removal of textiles quotas and the appreciation of the local currency resulted in decline in the sector's contribution during 2005. The third phase of AGOA in 2007 and the provision of rules of origin of third country have had implications on Lesotho's exports and employment of Basotho by the industry. The expiry of multi-fibre agreement (MFA) implied greater competition in the US market by more efficient countries such as China, also contributed to the problem. As a result, the ratio of textiles and clothing contribution to GDP declined from 9.2% in 2004 to 7.1% in 2005. Exports to the USA have also declined by 13% from 2004 to 2005 although there was a slight improvement from 2005 to 2006 of 2.2% [53]. These fluctuations invariably impacted on the Southern African Customs Union (SACU) revenue and the Lesotho economy, which relies on SACU revenue for most of its income (averaging 55%) [54].

The renegotiation of the SACU agreement and the revenue-sharing formula in the context of Free Trade Agreements (FTA) with the European Union (EU) and United States of America (USA) and the global financial crisis has led to a decline in customs revenues from M4.8 billion in 2009/2010 to about M2.3 billion in 2010/2011. This will mean a reduction in the Government's share in the economy.

3. Research methodology

The study area from which the data for this chapter is derived was comprised of all the textile and garment industry sites located in the districts of Maseru and Leribe. Prior to data collection exercise, the research protocol was submitted to the Lesotho Ministry of Health and Social Welfare Maseru, Ethics Review Committee, which reviewed and gave approval for the data collection. A multistage research design was used for data collection. First, a rapid appraisal questionnaire was administered to 38 factories from which 23 factories served as a sampling frame for the selection of six case study factories. Second, a factory workers' questionnaire, which was a cross-sectional survey instrument, was used to collect data from 640 factory workers among the six selected case-study firms. The number of factory workers interviewed was proportional to the number of workers in a factory. Research assistants were allowed into the factory premises during the lunch break hour, which is between 13.00 and 14.00 H. The original idea of randomly selecting workers for interviews prior to interview proved unworkable since researchers were not allowed access to the factory premises prior to lunch hour. Research assistants were allowed into the factory premises during lunch break to interview the workers. Nonetheless, the lowest response rate for the factories was 90%.

The quantitative data was analysed using descriptive and inferential statistics. Frequency tables were used to summarize pertinent information pertaining to key variables. Logistic regression analysis was employed to determine factors associated with the importance of employment provided by the industry and the likelihood of finding alternative work if retrenched. These analyses were performed using the Statistical Package for Social Sciences (SPSS). All ethical considerations such as confidentiality, informed consent and anonymity of subjects were strictly observed during data collection as well as analysis and dissemination of the findings.

4. Findings and discussion

4.1. Characteristics of firms and socio-demographics of the workers

Out of the 38 firms that received the rapid appraisal questionnaires, 2 firms declined to participate in the study. Of the remaining 36, only 23 completed their questionnaires and returned

http://dx.doi.org/10.5772/66653

them while 13 were outstanding giving a response rate of 64%. Attempts to follow up on the remaining questionnaires did not yield positive results. The selection of the study firms was, thus, based on 23 firms that responded to the appraisal questionnaire. Of the 23 firms that responded to the appraisal questionnaire six factories were selected as case study firms guided by three key criteria, namely, factory's exposure to: (1) economic globalization, in this case, focus was on perceived impact on trade and finance; (2) HIV and AIDS response, here the choice was guided by the type of response and the balance was preserved such that all types of responses (comprehensive, none and/or prevention only) were represented; and (3) production process type, whether firms specialise or engage in task shifting processes. **Table 2** presents the characteristics of these factories. From **Table 2**, it can be seen that all the factories were foreign owned with the exception of one. Half of the foreign-owned factories were South African followed by Taiwanese owned factories at 32%. About a tenth of the factories were Chinese owned while one factory was co-owned by Chinese, Taiwanese and other nationalities. Regarding the number of years that the factories have been operating in Lesotho, the result revealed that a fifth of the factories have been operating in Lesotho for 10 or more years while a third (35%) have been in Lesotho for between 5 and 9 years. Forty-four percent of the factories have been working in Lesotho for less than 5 years. There were disparities in the years of operation in Lesotho by factory ownership. Chinese factories have been in Lesotho longest with a mean of 12 years of operation followed by Taiwanese with a mean of 11 years, while the majority of South African factories have been in Lesotho for less than 5 years with a mean of 4 years of operation in Lesotho.

In addition, **Table 2** indicates that employment figures ranged from 260 to over 800 employees. Twenty-six percent of the factories had a workforce of between 500 and 799 followed by those with a workforce of less than 300 and those with a workforce of over 800 workers at 22% each. Workforce disparities were such that Taiwanese factories were employing 45% of the workforce followed by the South African factories with 37%. Chinese factories were employing 11% of the workforce while the other two factories employed 5% or less. Concerning trade patterns, **Table 2** further reveals that United States of America (USA) and the European Union (EU) are the main export destinations (39%) followed by the Southern African Customs Union (SACU) (17.4%) and the rest of the other export destinations constituted less than 10% of the exports. Seventeen percent of the factories were not exporting their products. Thus, the textiles and garment industry is more export oriented, hence more prone to the impact of economic globalization, preferential trade agreements and financial crisis that has hit the industry in recent times. The dominance of the Lesotho textiles industry by foreign firms has additional implications that the global economic crisis may affect the industry very hard due to demand for repatriation of profits abroad which will be affected by the economic crisis.

As regards sources of financial capital, 11 factories were financed from abroad while 8 were partly financed locally and partly from abroad. Only one factory was financed locally. Three factories did not provide information about their sources of financial capital. Of the 18 factories that provided information about the location of their financiers abroad, 44% were located in South Africa, 28% in Asia and 17% in the USA. Eleven percent of the factories had their foreign financiers situated in other countries than South Africa, Asia or the USA. From **Table 2**, 22 of 23 factories (96%) were foreign-owned companies, this coupled with the fact that about

Characteristic		Frequency	Percent
Factory ownership	Chinese	3	13.0
	Taiwanese	7	30.4
	South African	11	47.8
	Basotho	1	4.3
	Chinese + Taiwanese + Other	1	4.3
Years of operation in Lesotho	<5	10	43.5
	5–9	8	34.8
	10 +	5	21.7
	Mean		7.30
Factory employment size	< 300	5	21.7
	300-499	4	17.4
	500-799	6	26.1
	800 and above	5	21.7
	No response	3	13.0
Export destination	Do not export	4	17.4
	SACU	4	17.4
	SADC	2	8.7
	US & EU	9	39.1
	Other destinations	1	4.3
	SADC & US	1	4.3
	US, EU & OTHER	1	4.3
	No response	1	4.3

Table 2. Characteristics of the factories.

19 of the companies have their source of financing from abroad make the operations of the companies more dependent on the success of their operations in the international markets since most have foreign market destinations. Instability in the world economic market will hit these companies very hard unless the companies are well diversified to be able to absorb such a shock.

The distribution of the employees, as evidenced in **Table 3**, reveals that a quarter of the respondents were male compared to three quarters female (75%). Given the role of socialization and culture of the Basotho people that are more patriarchal, power relations and the gender dimensions of the labour force, both the women workforce and the operations of the factories may be at more risks of the HIV and AIDS epidemic unless more precautions and preventative measures are in place. To buttress this point, Hlalele and Letsie [37] posit that "women's minority status, religious and cultural beliefs and adverse economic conditions negatively

http://dx.doi.org/10.5772/66653

Characteristic	Frequency	Percent
Sex		
Male	158	24.7
Female	482	75.3
Experience of working at factories		
<2 years	238	37.2
2–3.99 years	207	32.3
4 years and above	188	29.4
No response	7	1.1
Age		
<20	14	2.2
20–24	118	18.4
25–29	188	29.4
30–34	138	21.6
35+	182	28.4
Educational attainment		
No education	14	2.2
Primary	269	42.0
Junior secondary	247	38.6
Senior secondary or better	110	17.2
Marital status		
Never married	169	26.4
Previous married	114	17.8
Currently married	355	55.5
No response/cohabiting	2	0.3
Total	**640**	**100.0**

Table 3. Some socio-demographic characteristics of the workers.

impact the health status of most Basotho women. This, therefore, makes it difficult for women to negotiate safer or protected sex within their relationships. As a consequence, women face increased chances of contracting sexually transmitted infections (STIs), HIV and AIDS and having undesired pregnancies. Gender-based violence and gender inequality are increasingly cited as important determinants of women's HIV risk." This calls for a stronger HIV and AIDS policy at the workplace and nationally to protect the workforce and women and ensuring sustainability of production. Slightly more than a third (37.2%) of the workforce had worked at the factories for less than 2 years, another third (32.3%) had been with the factories for 2 to less than 4 years and the remaining (29.4%) had worked at the factories for 4 years or more. Less than 5% of the respondents were less than 20 years old, majority (69%) were aged between 20 and 34 years and 28% were aged 35 years and above. Thus, about 70% or more of the workforce are 35 years of age or younger which places them within a more sexually active group with high risk of contracting HIV and AIDS at the workplace given unequal power relations between men and women when it comes to negotiating for protective sexual intercourse. Few (2%) of the workers had no formal education, while those with primary and junior secondary education were 42 and 40%, respectively. Less than 20% had senior secondary education or better. According to marital status, more than half (56%) of the workers were currently married compared to 26% who were never married and 18% previously married. This point bears very well on the socio-cultural dimension of the Basotho people, and at the workplace, as emphasised earlier by Hlalele and Letsie [37] who maintained that with more than 40% of the workforce unmarried, coupled with more patriarchal culture, younger women workforce with more possibility of intergenerational sex preference especially between older men and younger women may be driven by socio-economic conditions as a consequence of unequal power relations. This exposes the workforce to a much greater risk of HIV and AIDS infection detrimental to the workforce, the industry and the nation at large. The low level of educational attainment by the majority of the workforce, which is predominantly women, places the workers and by extension the women employees at more disadvantage in terms of power relations. This can further manifest itself in terms of low economic power and a target for intergenerational sex between older men and younger women with high risk of HIV and AIDS infection with a consequence of reduced productivity either due to sickness themselves or taking care of relatives who may also be infected or affected by the pandemic.

4.2. Economic empowerment

As indicated elsewhere in the chapter, PTAs have made it easier for Lesotho's products to have access to the USA and EU markets. According to results of the rapid appraisal information obtained from the managers and presented in **Table 4**, more than half (52%) of the workforce in the factories are employed by the factories that are exporting solely to the USA and the EU. Considering that some factories are exporting to the USA and or EU and other destinations, the percentage of the workforce employed as a result of the PTAs is over 60%. The success of the economic opportunities created by the PTAs is dependent on sustained market conditions under the economic globalization situation. Any economic instability in the global market can create serious repercussions as experienced during the 2008 global financial crisis which literally led to some of the factories closing down during the data collection phase of this study. Variation in exchange rate of the US$ and the South African Rand also impacts on the operations of the factories in Lesotho which often leads to threats of closure of the factories and loss of jobs. Thus, by implications, because women constitute over 70% of the workforce, they will be more affected and forced into more economic hardship. Besides, the factory job was the first job ever for majority of the women on account of their low level of education which made them not to find jobs in other sectors of the economy.

In assessing how the industry has benefited Basotho economically, the study found that 72% of the workers reported that their present job was their first job ever. Comparative figures were 77% for females and 57% for males and the difference between these percentages was

http://dx.doi.org/10.5772/66653

Export destination	Total employees	Percentage
Do not export	976	7
SACU	1612	11
SADC	536	4
US & EU	7458	52
Other destinations	501	4
SADC & US	1131	8
US & EU & other	1770	12
No response	242	2

Table 4. Distribution of employees by export destination.

statistically significant. Making it evident that the garment and textiles industry is making a positive difference by providing employment to Basotho who otherwise would be without jobs and this is more so among females than males. However, there were no salary differences between male and female employees. To further emphasize the importance of the jobs provided by the industry, of those workers for whom the present job was their first job ever, 81% were dependent on support from either parents or partners for those who were married. Only 5% were supporting themselves from agriculture. To further support the notion that females were benefiting more than their male counterparts, 66% of males compared to 86% of females were dependent on someone before being employed in the garment and textiles industry. In comparing present and previous salaries for those who had worked elsewhere prior to joining the firms, on the average, females were about M300 better off working in the industry while males were M40 worse off. Employment in the factories has enhanced women's economic empowerment and personal autonomy which of course could result into increased HIV vulnerability where there is unprotected sex depending on how the power relations is played out between the sexes following increased economic empowerment.

The logistic regression result in **Table 5** further lends support to the notion that economic opportunities of the garment and textiles industry are benefiting females more than males. The results of the logistic regression analysis indicate that males are less likely to have mentioned that the present job is their first ever implying that they joined the industry having previously worked elsewhere. This indicates that this sector appears to have created more job opportunities for women who previously had no job opportunities than for men. However, the results do confirm that females are the major beneficiaries of economic empowerment provided by the garment and textiles industry. This would not come as a surprise since Basotho men have always benefited from employment provided by the mining industry in South Africa. Recent retrenchments of Basotho men from the mines notwithstanding, mining work is still considered the best option among Basotho men. The logistic regression result also demonstrates that age is negatively associated with getting employment in the textiles and garment industry. One of the reasons why the Basotho males are less schooled than their female counterparts is due to the fact that education was not an important factor for getting

Variable		B	Exp(B)
Location	Maseru	0.265	1.304
	Leribe (RC)		
Sex	Male	−1.134**	0.322
	Female (RC)		
Age		−0.049**	0.952
Years of operation in Lesotho		−0.017	0.983
Type of work	Management	0.208	1.231
	Supervisor	-0.562	0.570
	Unskilled labourer	-0.194	0.824
	Skilled production worker (RC)		
Education	No education	0.350	1.419
	Junior secondary	0.215	1.240
	Senior secondary or better	0.310	1.363
	Primary (RC)		
Marital status	Never married	0.460#	1.584
	Previously married	−0.163	0.850
	Currently married		
Sub-sector	Knitting garments	−0.130	0.878
	Denim/cotton yarn	−0.494#	0.610
	Woven garments (RC)		
Production process	Specialisation and division of labour	0.302	1.352
	Multi-skilling and task shifting (RC)		
Constant		2.706**	

Notes: $^{**}p < 1\%$; $^{*}p < 5\%$ and $^{\#}$ $p < 10\%$.

Table 5. Logistic regression results showing the odds that the current job is the first ever.

a mining job. History would seem to be repeating itself in the textiles and garment industry where education is not an important factor for the industry providing one with the first job ever. It would seem sex and age are the main factors associated with the odds that the present job is the first ever. Marital status and subsector are marginally associated with the odds that the present job is the first ever.

4.3. Threats to economic opportunities

The economic opportunities provided by the industry's jobs are threatened by several factors, both external and internal. For purposes of this chapter, however, only two factors (HIV and

AIDS and economic globalization) were taken into consideration. It is common for firms to cut salaries when … for self-ill-health workers are absent from work due to self-ill-health. Ninety-one percent of the workers reported that there are salary cuts when they are absent due to ill-health. Over 80% of the workers also reported that absence from work due to reasons other than ill-health attracts salary cuts. Given the high HIV prevalence in Lesotho and among the workers of the industry in particular with more than 40% prevalence rate [49], workers are bound to be away from work because they are either sick themselves or they have to look after sick relatives. On a typical month, the workers are on the average away from work for 6.34 days which is astonishingly high. Salary cuts should be understood in the context where employers have to replace absent workers by temporary staff in order to meet the deadlines of their orders. Absenteeism due to ill-health also impacts on the employers in terms of lost time or having to deal with substitute casual workers whose productivity may be lower than that of regular employees whom they are replacing.

Women are known to be half of the world's migrants and also half of those living with HIV and AIDS [12, 20] and labour migration and other forms of mobility have been associated with increased risk to HIV infection [55, 56]. However, most of the female migrant workers are from the rural mountainous areas of Lesotho. Although most of the respondents were from these areas, there was no indication that there was a breakdown in relationships and the formation of long-term relationships at the factories as has been shown by some studies [55]. This is because most of the women respondents (56%) were married though many stated that they rarely visit home to meet their spouses. Kendall and Pelcastre [55] echoed that internal migration involves the processes of rupture and reformation of social networks. However, there was no evidence pertaining to this in this research. Nonetheless, it can be argued that some migrants apart from the continued economic responsibilities for themselves and their dependents, who have pushed people away from their homes to seek work in the factories, do escape from home community and/or family controls and potential isolation back at home.

It is a widely held view that social vulnerability of poverty contributes to workers, especially women, to the risk of HIV infection [16, 37, 57]. For example, in the context of South Africa, Gilbert and Selikow [58] argue that the HIV epidemic in South Africa and the region at large is increasingly feminized as a growing proportion of new infections occur among women and affect women. It is revealed that in South Africa, a perilous mix of biomedical, political, economic and cultural forces shape the gendered dynamic of the HIV epidemic. The vulnerability can also be attributed to male partners' sexual infidelity having concurrent and multiple sexual partnerships and the lack of condom use which exemplify the link between internal migration and HIV vulnerability and not just international migration which has been the focus of many studies. Therefore, this chapter confirms Webber's [59] assertion that women's biological as well as their social vulnerabilities to the pandemic may be exacerbated within the context of international labour migration and rural-urban migration [4]. The scourge of HIV and AIDS is a complex, multifaceted issue that requires a collaborative effort and hence multidimensional strategies.

The second threat to economic opportunities offered by factory work is global economic crisis. The recent food prices instability on the international market have been at the centre of debates and as Galtier [60] maintains, experts have described the situation in the late 2000s in developing countries as one that is characterized by instability in food prices. One of the causes is globalization which Galtier [60] calls imported instability. Using qualitative design, Uraguchi [61] conducted a study on farming households in Bangladesh and Ethiopia which focused on the vulnerability of women to food insecurity owing to the 2007–2008 food price hikes and their seasonal coping mechanisms. The study confirms that it is gender inequality that makes women more vulnerable to the food price hikes, yet they are resourcefully devising ways to cope with scarcity, access and consumption of food. Women remain highly vulnerable to external shocks and they have fragile intra-household coping mechanisms. In this current study, 91% of the workers who were aware of the global economic crisis reported that the global economic crisis was likely to bring about retrenchment and more economic hardship for them and their families. The economic crisis posed significant threats to the developing countries. Gaerlan et al. [62] argue that global economic crisis has fuelled the continuing job insecurity through "casualisation" in the Philippines, and this has caused women to change their lifestyles by letting go non-essential goods and services. Reductions in employment in the formal economy and escalating food and fuel prices are forcing more and more people into the informal economy as the viable option [63]. In this study, the impact of the global economic crisis has threatened loss of jobs among women employees especially on account of their low level of education with the current job being their first job ever for most of the women. Cohen [63] reports that female traders are insecure and vulnerable since they are earning incomes that are insufficient for supporting a household, reinvesting in their business or saving money. Horn [64] maintains that incomes and employment trend for women in the informal sector are increasing vulnerability and women struggle more to feed their families through cutting back on educational and medical expenses. The women employed in the textile and garment industry in Lesotho were no exception despite the fact that the result of the data analysis revealed women were better off than men from their jobs in the textiles industry. In another study, Mutekwa [65] demonstrated that the discourses of the African renaissances are entangled in the gendered and gendering nature of globalisation discourse since they are framed within it. The study further identified the multifaceted implications and effects of a hegemonic, masculine neoliberal global discourse on the various facets of the African Renaissance concluding that the African Renaissances responses can be either complicit or subversive in addressing key challenges in a globalizing economy with gender sensitivity.

Women and ethnic minority workers have been particularly hard hit, not just by job losses but also by reductions in hours of work, wage rates and non-wage benefits [66]. Similar findings have been documented on the impact of the global crisis on workers in many countries [67–69]. The conundrum even more worrying is that 61% of these workers opined that they are not likely to get a job should they be retrenched due to low level of education and non-availability of jobs. According to the logistic regression results in **Table 6**, age is the only major explanatory variable from the perception of the workers that they would not get a job if retrenched. Education is a marginal explanatory variable except that in factories, the perception of the workers that the likelihood of getting a job if retrenched is low due to low level of education. The poor educational level of participants can be attributed to the difficult economic situation which has truncated their educational opportunities. However, the factories

http://dx.doi.org/10.5772/66653

Variable		B	Exp(B)
Sex	Male	0.288	1.334
	Female		
Age		−0.072**	0.931
Type of work done	Management	−0.668	0.513
	Supervisor	−0.635	0.530
	Unskilled labourer	−0.243	0.784
	Skilled production worker (RC)		
Education	No education	−1.118#	0.327
	Junior secondary	−0.129	0.879
	Senior secondary or better	0.308	1.361
	Primary		
Marital status	Never married	0.349	1.418
	Previously married	0.277	1.319
	Currently married		
Sub-sector	Knitting garment	−0.239	0.788
	Denim fabric/cotton yarn	−0.420	0.657
	Woven garment (RC)		
Years of operation in Lesotho		−0.018	0.982
Number of employees		0.000	1.000
Absence due to ill health	No	−0.234	0.792
	Yes (RC)		
Constant		2.931**	

Notes: **$p < 1\%$; *$p < 5\%$ and # $p < 10\%$.

Table 6. The perceived likelihood of finding alternative work if retrenched.

organize on-the-job training of their semi-skilled employees who easily fit into the production line jobs but due to their low level of education, once retrenched from the factories may not easily get jobs elsewhere.

Furthermore, the findings show that the economic opportunities provided by the industry do not appear to go beyond employment provision. Asked whether they provided employee benefits such as housing, medical aid, funeral cover, pension and life insurance as one way of empowering their workers, employers indicated that they do not provide benefits to their employees with the exception of employees in clerical and management positions. As Pelcastre-Villafuerte et al. [70] aptly put it, the family responsibilities make low-wage factory work the most viable option for women, though these jobs are sometimes without legally mandated medical and social security benefits associated with them. However, the industry does provide minimal benefits stipulated in the labour code.

5. Conclusion and recommendations

The textiles and garment industry attracts a huge number of workers, especially women from the rural mountainous areas of Lesotho who would otherwise be unemployed. This has greatly been as a result of Lesotho enjoying PTAs from the USA and EU. Although the employment of these rural female migrants in this industry provides economic opportunities and economically empowers them, there are challenges posed by both external and internal forces such as the global economic crisis as well as the HIV and AIDS pandemic.

The challenge posed by the global economic crisis has created a sense of job insecurity among workers with 61% of these workers having opined that they are not likely to get a job should they be retrenched due to low level of education. The study found that age was the only major explanatory variable from the perception of the workers that they would not get a job if retrenched. Education is a marginal explanatory variable except that in factories, the perception of the workers that the likelihood of getting a job if retrenched is low due to low level of education. This study also established that it was a common practice for firms in the textile and garment industry in Lesotho to cut salaries whenever workers are absent from work irrespective of whether such absence is due to ill-health. Ninety-one percent of the workers reported that there are salary cuts when they are absent due to ill-health. Over 80% of the workers also reported that absence from work due to reasons other than ill-health attracts salary cuts. Given the high HIV prevalence in Lesotho and among the workers of the industry in particular with more than 40% prevalence rate [49], workers are bound to be away from work because they are either sick themselves or they have to look after sick relatives.

The study also revealed that 75% of the labour force in the industry is made of women as major beneficiaries of employment opportunities although most of them are in their sexually active age (25–39 years old) with unequal gender power relations which make them more vulnerable to the threat posed by the HIV/AIDS pandemic as double-edged sword. This was inferred from the high prevalence rate (43%) of HIV/AIDS infection in the industry with women having prevalence rate of 44% compared to men at 35%. This has major ramifications for sustainability of the industry in both the perspective of the workers and firms without any major policy in place to curb the spread of the HIV/AIDS. Thus, the combined effect of the global economic crisis and the HIV/AIDS pandemic coupled with unequal gender relations in the industry make women more vulnerable than their male counterparts. This outcome is in agreement with a number of authors who identified gender inequality as a major driver for the spread of HIV and AIDS [8, 39–42]. Similar views were expressed by Epstein et al. [43] and Mitchell et al. [44] who claim that gender inequalities fuel HIV and AIDS pandemic and make women more vulnerable to infection. Nonetheless, the opportunities offered by the industry do not go beyond the provision of employment as many workers do not enjoy social insurance and other benefits. Any further retrenchment from this industry would have serious negative

http://dx.doi.org/10.5772/66653

impact not only on the economy as a whole but on individual workers and their families since the South African mines have increasingly been retrenching workers, especially foreign-based workers which the Basotho form the majority.

The Department of Labour and Employment has not been able to follow-up with HIV and AIDS responses by the industry neither has it also insisted on various fringe benefits that should accrue to the workers. There is too much reliance by the Government of Lesotho on this industry to provide the necessary jobs at this time of the global economic crisis. The industry is kept afloat because of external capital flow and the end of PTAs can be catastrophic for the government and Basotho and as such dash their hopes for a better economy and decent lives.

The government should invest in diversification of employment opportunities, especially as Lesotho is blessed with abundant natural resources such as mohair and wool, mineral resources and water among many others. Although the Government of Lesotho is already doing much in the area of HIV and AIDS, the Department of Labour and Employment needs to ensure that all factories comply with its stipulations vis-à-vis HIV and AIDS response within the workplace. Also, the department should strive to encourage all the factories to institute fringe benefits not only to a selected few, especially expatriates as is the present case. This gesture needs to be extended to all workers.

Author details

Pius Tangwe Tanga[1]*, Haruna M. Bello[2], Tiisetso J. Makatjane[3] and Tumelo Tsikoane[4]

*Address all correspondence to: ptanga@ufh.ac.za

1 Department of Social Work/Social Development, University of Fort Hare, South Africa

2 Department of Agricultural Economics, University of Namibia, Mandume Ndemufayo Avenue, Winhoek, Namibia

3 Department of Statistics and Demography, National University of Lesotho, Lesotho

4 Department of Development Studies, National University of Lesotho, Lesotho

References

[1] Bello HM, Tsikoane T, Mochebelele M, Tanga PT, Nchake M, Makatjane TJ, Letete J. Economic Globalisation-HIV and AIDS-Nexus in the Textile and Garment Industry in Lesotho (unpublished). Maseru: National University of Lesotho; 2010.

[2] Bureau of Statistics. 2006 Lesotho Population and Housing Census Analytical Report, Volume IIIB Socio Economic Characteristics. Maseru: Bureau of Statistics; 2009.

[3] National AIDS Commission. Report on the National Response to HIV and AIDS (Period: 2006–2010). Maseru: National AIDS Commission; 2010.

[4] Tanga PT, Tangwe MN. The interplay between economic empowerment and HIV and AIDS amongst migrant workers in the textile industry in Lesotho. SAHARA-J: Journal of Social Aspects of HIV/AIDS: An Open Access Journal. 2014; 11 (1): 187–201. DOI:10.1080/17290376.2014.976250.

[5] United Nations Statistics Division. Lesotho Country Responses to HIV/AIDS Prevention. [Internet].2010. Available from: http://www.indexmundi.com/lesotho/hiv-prevention.html [Accessed: 2015/12/10].

[6] UNICEF. Revised country programme document: Lesotho (2008–2012). Maseru: UNICEF; 2007.

[7] UNAIDS. Uniting the World against AIDS. [Internet]. 2009. Available from: http://www.unaids.org/en/CountryResponses/Countries/lesotho.asp. [Accessed: 2012/10/9].

[8] Tanga, PT. The impact of declining extended family support system on the education of orphans in Lesotho. African Journal of AIDS Research. 2013; 12(3):173–183.

[9] Com Mark Trust: Apparel Lesotho Alliance to Fight Aids; 2007. Available from: http//:www.commark.org/pages/Default.asp?SectionID=182. [Accessed 2014/10/23].

[10] Bureau of Statistics. Provisional 2006 Population Figures. Maseru: Bureau of Statistics; 2008.

[11] Ministry of Health and Social Welfare (MOHSW). Lesotho Demographic and Health Survey 2009. Maseru, Lesotho: MOHSW; 2010.

[12] UNAIDS. Report of the global AIDS epidemic. [Internet]. 2008. Available from: http://www.unaids.org/en/KnowledgeCentre/HIVData/GlobalReport/2008/2008_Global_Report.asp. [Accessed 2012/2/12].

[13] Central Bank of Lesotho. Annual Report. Maseru: Central Bank of Lesotho; 2006.

[14] Bureau of Statistics. 2006 Lesotho Population and Housing Census Analytical Report, Volume IIIA Population Dynamics. Maseru: Bureau of Statistics; 2009.

[15] Metcalfe BD, Rees CJ. Gender, globalization and organization: exploring power, relations and intersections. Equality, diversity and Inclusion: International Journal. 2010; 29 (1): 5–22.

[16] Townsend L, Giorgio M, Zembe Y, Cheyip M, Mathews C. HIV Prevalence and Risk Behaviour Among Foreign Migrant Women Residing in Cape Town, South Africa. AIDS Behaviour, Online publication. 2014. DO 10.1007/s10461-014-0784-1.

[17] Altman D. Aids and the globalization of sexuality. Journal of Social Identities. 2008; 14 (2):146–147.

[18] Sapkota JB. Mainstreaming globalization in poverty reduction strategy papers in the Asia-Pacific region. Development in Practice. 2011; 21 (7): 999–1012

[19] Altman D: Sexuality and globalization. Agenda. 2004; 1(62): 22–28.

[20] Hirsch JS. Review: labour migration, externalities and ethics: theorizing the meso-level determinants of HIV vulnerability. Social Science & Medicine. 2014; 100: 38–45.

[21] Pearson R. Moving the goalposts: gender and globalization in the twenty-first century. Gender and Development. 2000; 8(1): 10–19.

[22] Sen G. Globalization in the 21st century: challenges for civil society. University of Amsterdam Development Lecture. Available from the Institute for Development Research Amsterdam (IDRA), University of Amsterdam, Plantage Muidergracht 12, 1018 TV Amsterdam, The Netherlands.

[23] Bureau of Statistics. 2002/03 and 1994/95 Household Budget Survey Analytical Report Volume 1. Maseru: Bureau of Statistics; 2006.

[24] Ministry of Health and Social Welfare [MOHSW], ICF Macro. Lesotho Demographic and Health Survey 2009. Maseru, Lesotho: MOHSW and ICF Macro; 2010.

[25] African Development Bank [ADB]. Kingdom of Lesotho—2008-2012 Country Strategic Paper. Maseru: ADB; 2008.

[26] UNPD. Human Development Report. Geneva: UNDP; 2009.

[27] United Nations Children's Fund [UNICEF]. The State of the World's Children 20118. New York: UNICEF; 2011.

[28] Bureau of Statistics. Consumer Price Index: Statistical Reports No. 19: 2011. Maseru: Bureau of Statistics; 2011.

[29] Bureau of Statistics. National Accounts of Lesotho 1999–2008: Statistical Reports No. 32: 2009. Maseru: Bureau of Statistics; 2009.

[30] Lesotho Review. An Overview of Kingdom of Lesotho's Economy. Maseru, Lesotho: Central Bank of Lesotho; 2008.

[31] National AIDS Commission: National HIV and AIDS Policy. Maseru, Lesotho: National AIDS Commission; 2007.

[32] Government of Lesotho [GOL]. Revised National HIV & AIDS Strategic Plan 2006–2011. Maseru, LS: NAC; 2009.

[33] National AIDS Commission, UNAIDS, Family Health International. Gender and Multiple and Concurrent Sexual Partnerships in Lesotho. Maseru: National AIDS Commission; 2009.

[34] Camlin CS, Kwena ZA, Dworkin SL, Cohen CR, Bukusi EA. She mixes her business: HIV transmission and acquisition risks among female migrants in western Kenya. Social Science & Medicine. 2013, 102: 146–156.

[35] Curtis S. Health and Inequality—Geographical Perspectives. London: Sage; 2004.

[36] Meade MS, Earickson RJ. Medical Geography. 2nd edition. New York/London: The Guilford Press; 2000.

[37] Hlalele D, Letsie PR. Gender Inequality and HIV/AIDS in Lesotho: a human disease ecological perspective. Journal of Human Ecology. 2011; 36(3): 159–165.

[38] Nattrass N. Gender access to antiretroviral treatment in South Africa. Feminist Economics. 2008; 14(4): 19–36.

[39] Poku N. Poverty, debt and Africa's HIV/AIDS crisis. International Affairs. 2002; 78: 531–546.

[40] Natrass N. The Moral Economy of AIDS in South Africa. Cape Town: Cambridge; 2004.

[41] Braun YA, Dreiling MC. From developmentalism to HIV/AIDS crisis: the amplification of women's rights in Lesotho. International Feminist Journal of Politics. 2010; 12(3–4): 464–483.

[42] Hatcher A, de Wet J, Bonell CP, Strange V, Phetla G. Promoting critical consciousness and social mobilisation in HIV/AIDS programmes: lessons and curricular tools from a South African intervention. Health Education Research. 2011; 26(3):542–555.

[43] Epstein D, Morell R, Moletsane R, Unterhalter E. Gender and HIV/AIDS in Africa south of the Sahara: interventions, activism, identities. Transformation: Critical Perspectives on Southern Africa. 2004; 54: 1–16.

[44] Mitchell S, Cockroft A, Lamothe G, Anderson N. Equity in HIV testing: evidence from cross-sectional study in ten Southern African countries. BMC International Health and Human Rights. 2010; 10: 23–33.

[45] Poulsen H. The gendered impact of HIV/AIDS on education in South Africa and Swaziland: save the children's experiences. Gender and Development. 2006; 14 (1): 47–56.

[46] Bajaj M. Sugar daddies and the dangers of sugar: cross-generational relationships, HIV/AIDS, and secondary schooling in Zambia. In David PB, Alexander WW (eds). Gender, Equality and Education from International and Comparative Perspectives (International Perspectives on Education and Society). West Yorkshire: Emerald Group Publishing Limited; 2009, 10: 123–143.

[47] Mindry D. Engendering care: HIV, humanitarian assistance in Africa and the reproduction of gender stereotypes. Culture, Health & Sexuality. 2010; 12(5): 555–568.

[48] Jewkes R. Where to for sexual health education for adolescents in Sub-Saharan Africa? PLoS Med. 2010; 7(6): e10000288. Doi: 10.1371/journal.pmed.10000288.

[49] ALAFA. Lesotho Apparel Industry Unites to Fight AIDS. Maseru: ALAFA; 2009.

[50] Bennet M. Lesotho's export textile and garment industry. In Jauch H, Traub-Merz (eds). The Future of the Textile and Clothing Industry in Sub-Saharan Africa. Bonn: Friedrich-Ebert-Stiftung; 2006.

[51] Lesotho Review. An Overview of Kingdom of Lesotho's Economy; 2007 edition.

[52] Kim J-O, Traore MK, Warfield C. The textile and apparel industry in developing countries. Textile Progress. 2006; 38 (3): 1–64.

[53] Central Bank of Lesotho. The phasing out of the IMF—Fibre Agreement (MFA): its implications on Lesotho. Economic Review. 2005.

[54] Masenyetse RF, Motelle SI. Government Revenue—expenditure nexus in Lesotho: the decline in SACU revenue. American Journal of Economics. 2012; 2 (1): 8–14.

[55] Kandell T, Pelcastre BE. HIV vulnerability and condom use among migrant workers in Puebla, Mexico. Health Care for Women International. 2010; 31: 515–532.

[56] Jordal M, Wijewardena K, Öhman A, Essen B, Olsson P. Negotiating respectability: migrant women workers' perceptions of relationships and sexuality in free trade zones in Sri Lanka. Health Care for Women International. 2014, 35 (6): 658–676.

[57] Connelly P, Rosen S. Will small and medium enterprises provide HIV and AIDS services to employees? An analysis of market demand. South African Journal of Economics. 2005; 73: 613–626

[58] Gilbert L, Selikow TA. The epidemic in this country has the face of a woman: gender and HIV/AIDS in South Africa. African Journal of Aids Research. 2011; 10 (supplement): 325–334.

[59] Webber G. The impact of migration on HIV prevention for women: constructing a conceptual framework. Health Care for Women International. 2008; 28: 712–731.

[60] Galtier F. Which instruments best tackle food price instability in developing countries? Development in Practice, 2011; 21 (4–5): 526–535.

[61] Uraguchi ZW. Food price hike, food security and gender equality: assessing the roles and vulnerability of women in households of Bangladesh and Ethiopia. Gender and Development. 2010; 18(3): 491–501.

[62] Gaerlan K, Cabrera M, Samla P, Santoalla L. Feminised recession: impact of the global financial crisis on women garment workers in the Philippines. Gender and Development. 2010; 18(2): 229–240.

[63] Cohen J. How the global economic crisis reaches marginalised workers: the case of street traders in Johannesburg, South Africa. Gender and Development. 2010; 18(2): 277–289.

[64] Horn EZ. The effects of global crisis on women in the informal economy: research findings from WIEGO and the Inclusive Cities partners. Gender and Development. 2010; 18(2): 263–276.

[65] Mutekwa A. Gendered globalization discourses: implications for the African Renaissance. International Journal of African Renaissance Studies. 2012; 7(1): 5–21.

[66] Lawson M, King R. If not now, when? [Internet]. 2008. Available from: http:www.oxfam.org.uk/resources/policy/debt_aid/downloads/bn. g20summit%20.pdf [Accessed 2010/2/24].

[67] Arguello R. Securing the fruits of their labours: the effect of the crisis on women in Peru's Ica Valley. Gender and Development. 2010; 18(2): 241–247.

[68] Fernandez B. Cheap and disposable? The impact of the global economic crisis on the migration of Ethiopian women domestic workers to the Gulf. Gender and Development. 2010; 18(2): 249–262.

[69] Espey J, Harper C, Jones N. Crisis, care and childhood: the impact of economic crisis on care work in poor households in the developing world. Gender and Development. 2010; 18(2): 291–307.

[70] Pelcastre-Villafuerte B, Kandell T, Magis C. Las maquiladoras frente al VIH/AIDS, implementacion de programas y percepcion de los empleadores en Puebla. Region y sociedad. 2008; 20 (43): 189–211.